W9-BAF-597

WHAT DID YOU SAY?

An Unexpected Journey into the World of Hearing Loss
Second Edition

WHAT DID YOU SAY?

*An Unexpected Journey
into the World of Hearing Loss*
Second Edition

Monique E. Hammond

Two Harbors Press

Copyright © 2016 by Monique E. Hammond.

Two Harbors Press
322 First Avenue N, 5th floor
Minneapolis, MN 55401
612.455.2293
www.TwoHarborsPress.com

All rights reserved. No part of this publication may be reproduced, stored in a
retrieval system, or transmitted, in any form or by any means, electronic, mechanical,
photocopying, recording, or otherwise, without the prior written permission of the
author.

ISBN-13: 978-1-63413-828-4
LCCN: 2015921277

Distributed by Itasca Books

Cover Design by Jill Kennedy
Typeset by Jaime Willems
All diagrams by Monique E. Hammond unless otherwise indicated.

Printed in the United States of America

This book is not a medical textbook or a diagnostic reference book. The book is based on the author's own experience with sudden hearing loss and equilibrium problems. The narrative is for background information only. Although it is not all-inclusive, the information is correct to the best knowledge of the author.

This book does not dispense medical advice and does not advocate or sanction self-diagnosis and self-treatment. The author does not endorse any specific products, treatments, or medications. People with ear and/or hearing-related issues should seek prompt medical advice from appropriate physicians and health professionals. Responsibility for harm or damage resulting from a failure to do so does not rest with the author. The contents of this book are not to be used as reference in legal cases.

Contents

CONTENTS

PART FIVE
ASSISTIVE LISTENING DEVICES; ASL; SPEECH READING

PART SIX
SURGICAL IMPLANTS

PART SEVEN
FEELINGS and EMOTIONS, SUPPORT GROUPS, and ORGANIZATIONS

APPENDIX

Checklists

INTRODUCTION

Ever since the first edition of this book was printed, the world of hearing loss has become a lot more crowded. By now, one in five Americans, age twelve and over, have enough hearing loss to interfere with communication. Noise-induced hearing loss is on a sharp rise, especially among younger people. Researchers are trying to find ways to "fix" hearing loss with gene and stem cell therapies. Hearing aids are becoming ever more sophisticated, and many of the implants are getting a major electronic make-over. Among such flurries of activity, let's hope that the message of *prevention* will not be lost. That said, a lot has happened, and I feel that it is important to share some of those details with you in the second edition of this book.

But, back to the beginning...

This is the story of my sudden hearing loss. I am still trying to comprehend how, within a few short hours, my life was totally turned upside down. I suddenly was deaf in my left ear and my right one felt awfully stressed. I had balance problems and the injured ear began to buzz and hiss. I ended up in the hospital in dire straits. This all came as a total shock. My hearing had been my keenest sense. To this day, I am not sure exactly what happened. Until I came down with ear problems, however, I had taken my hearing for granted, just like everybody else.

Within the world of hearing loss, I have joined the ranks of the hard-of-hearing (HOH) people. We live in an oral communication gray zone. Although we are not deaf, we are challenged to varying degrees by different types of hearing loss.

I wrote this book in order to pass forward what I learned about hearing loss and its consequences as I tried to learn to deal with my own condition. Access to some organized, easy-to-understand information related to ear and hearing issues would have been enormously helpful to me in those early days. At the outset, I was surprised that I had problems asking precise and meaningful questions of the specialists who cared for me. After all, I had spent my professional life as a hospital pharmacist. I had a good understanding of the anatomy and function of the ears and of the many conditions that can befall them. I knew plenty about ear infections and their treatments. I was familiar with ototoxic, or ear-poisonous, medications. I was no stranger to inner ear-related dizziness, which brings people frequently to the emergency room. My knowledge, however, was spotty at best in specialized areas like audiology, hearing aids, assistive listening devices and conditions that frequently accompany hearing loss. Information that I gleaned from discussions with professionals left me with more questions than answers. I learned that vague questions get vague answers, although to be fair, there often were no clear-cut answers to be had. I determined eventually that even specialists had trouble navigating the murky waters of hearing loss. After a while, it became obvious that I had to do the investigating myself if I wanted to make sense out of my case.

As I searched for documentation, I found plenty of disjointed bits and pieces but nothing that painted a whole picture of the incident and of its eventual repercussions. By backtracking the events, tying up loose ends, and filling in knowledge gaps, I wrote this book—one that would have been helpful to me. I feel that I have created a systematic core of material that can serve any who live in the confusing world of hearing loss. I also hope to provide some useful insights to those who want to learn more so that they can help a loved one who struggles with hearing loss and its related challenges.

My story is certainly not all-inclusive. It does not cover everything that is known or important about hearing and ears. It is not meant to dispense medical advice or to assist in self-diagnosis, and in that respect, I issue a word of caution: people who experience any kind of ear- or hearing-related symptoms *must consult their physician or ear specialist for proper diagnosis and treatment.* For this account, the names of health care professionals were changed.

I hope this book provides you with enough background details to help you ask concise questions and to have informed discussions with your doctors and hearing specialists. I also hope that it encourages you to become involved in your own care, to persevere, and to insist on answers that are understandable to you.

PART ONE
MY STORY

CHAPTER 1
The Day Life Changed Forever

By profession I am a hospital pharmacist. Until that fateful Monday, which I came to call D-Day, I also enjoyed teaching. On a lovely fall afternoon, I met a new group of students for the start of their required pharmacology course. Things did not bode well. It seemed like we had the worst room in the whole building. It was uninviting, too small, and dark, with an acute shortage of chairs. We borrowed additional seating from the break room across the hall and rearranged the tables. There was certainly not much space for spreading out, but eventually we settled in. We had a somewhat choppy start, to say the least, but it got worse.

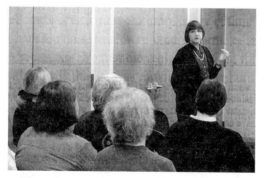

The author teaching a class *photo: R.Hammond*

The first chapter in the course book dealt with basic math, a fact that annoyed some of the students, although it was a requirement for the hands-on health profession that these young people had chosen. Class began at 3:00 p.m. It became immediately obvious that the adverse feelings of a few would make for a rather stressful afternoon. In hindsight, something was already brewing in my head, and the added pressure put me over the top.

About halfway through the session, I noticed that the hearing in my left ear clouded over. Guppy-mouth movements failed to pop it. I did not have any pain or any other symptoms, and I wondered if I was coming down with a cold.

I continued to teach the class, never missing a beat, even as my hearing gradually faded away, but I became increasingly worried. Was I having a stroke? I had no tingling or numbness of the face, no memory loss, no headache, no dizziness—nothing. So why was my hearing in free fall? Although I had trouble locating sound, I was able to respond to all student questions by relying on my right ear.

By 7:00 p.m., the end of the class period, my ear felt as if it were stuffed with cotton; it was totally deaf. Yet I remained amazingly calm—people who experience shock often seem to react that way. If anybody had come to me and described a similar episode, I would have advised that person to immediately hurry to the emergency room, but I could not think straight on my own behalf. I decided that I would call the doctor's office in the morning and insist on a same-day appointment.

By the time Ross, my husband, picked me up at school, it felt like life was chugging along in slow motion. My reactions had become sluggish, and I was quite tired. As I got into the car, I mentioned sort of casually that I was half-deaf and that I would have to see the physician about this rather scary development. Ross wondered if we should go to the hospital, but I declined. I had no pain and no fever. It could all wait until morning. We went home and I managed to fix dinner for us. I also left a message on the school program director's voice mail, explaining that we needed a bigger and better classroom. By 10:00 p.m., I was ready for bed. Then, as soon as my head hit the pillow, the room began to whirl around and around and would not stop. I became violently ill. My husband remarked that he felt fine; there hadn't been anything wrong with the food we'd had for supper. I hardly had the strength to talk. "It's not my stomach," I whispered. "It's my ear." Again, Ross suggested that we should go to the emergency room. I countered that the nausea would have to settle down first. Looking back, I still cannot believe how incredibly clouded my judgment was.

As I lay on the bathroom floor, hugging the toilet, the pieces of the puzzle fell gradually into place, and a very dark and devastating reality set in. I had been experiencing popping noises in that ear and an overall queasiness for almost two weeks. These turned out to be signs of the destructive forces that bore down on my left inner ear. Although I did not realize it at the time, life was about to change forever.

CHAPTER 2
My Last Days as a Fully Hearing Person

Two weeks before D-Day, my husband and I went on a marvelous Alaskan cruise. I had always wanted to see that last frontier, as it is one of the places that rates highly on the "bucket list"—sites to see before one dies.

Ah, the views—there is nothing quite like it. The fall colors set the tundra aglow, and the mountaintops looked as if they had been dusted with powdered sugar by the first high-altitude snowfalls. In anticipation of the approaching winter many animals had begun their slow descent down the slopes, heading to the milder conditions of the valleys.

As with most travel expeditions, the trip proved to be a health-risk disaster. But who thinks of all that when one is having a great time? Taxis, planes, trains, buses, hotels, and confined spaces on the ship itself were all germ havens. Plenty of noise, altitude variations, and climate changes became naturally part of the vacation experience. As the doctor mentioned later on, the trek was a perfect set-up for catching a viral infection or for aggravating an existing one.

My tourist enthusiasm became dampened by occasional popping noises in my left ear. They seemed to flare up in response to pressure changes inside my head. When the bus made the uphill climb in Denali Park or whenever I yawned, another round of these pesky, dull sounds unsettled me. Might they be middle-ear muscle spasms? Except for wondering about allergies or an oncoming cold, I had no explanation for the thumping. I reacted every time by pressing my thumb against the lower portion of the ear and along the jaw line, and every time the pressure brought on tenderness—no pain, just tenderness. This alarmed me, and I made a mental note to see the doctor promptly when we got home. At the time, I had little appreciation for the fact that something was going desperately wrong with that left ear.

I am relatively tolerant to the motions of the sea, unless the waves get really rolling. My husband is the one who strikes a stomach-grabbing pose at the mere sight of any water transportation. To my amazement, however, I was the one who felt queasy and mildly unwell as we sailed the very calm waters of Alaska's Inside Passage. I thought maybe I had eaten something that did not agree with me, but I could not pinpoint what the offensive food might have been. Looking back, this should have been a huge red flag that pointed to inner-ear trouble. Ross was just fine as we cruised along, while I went in search of seasickness relief. The medication that was handed to me at the reception desk was called, appropriately, "Sea Calm." It made me tired, and I slept most of the afternoon. After that, I felt all right for the rest of the trip, except for the annoying ear popping. Although I did not realize it, a storm was gathering—not on the waters outside but deep inside my head, in the bony cavities that house the delicate structures of the hearing and balance systems.

I was called in to work as soon as we got home, and so I neglected to contact the doctor's office. The thumping had let up by this time, and the fact that I did not have any pain or a fever eased my sense of urgency. Like so many health complaints, I thought that maybe the problem had fixed itself.

***

On Sunday, three days after our return from Alaska, we took my mother-in-law to a church fund-raiser. The exhilarating ethnic tunes, intended to fire up the giving spirits of the audience, would have been enjoyable, had they not been so offensively loud. We arrived just in time for the Greek selections. The amplifiers blasted the cafeteria-sized hall with mind-numbing sound. The music, punctuated by enthusiastic screams from the crowd, became so agonizingly intense that little children ran around covering their ears, trying to flee the scene. I should have joined them.

In the buffet line, patrons merely pointed at their food choices. I screamed to one server that such a racket could easily cause hearing damage—the longer the exposure, the greater the danger. Might he mention this to the amplifier fanatic? The man just stared at me, and I realized he probably could not hear me at all. Too much noise.

As we sat down to eat, my left ear was turned toward the stage with the sound blasters, a fact that the doctor later felt had been a significant contributor to my woes. Under the circumstances, a family conversation was impossible. We inhaled our lunch and left. On the way home, my left ear crackled off and on and felt somewhat dull.

CHAPTER 3
D-Day and Beyond

On Monday, the day after the fund-raiser, my world caved in. This was the Monday of the grueling 3:00-to-7:00 p.m. pharmacology class; the Monday when I spent several nighttime hours lying on the bathroom floor, miserably ill.

As midnight approached, I still could not even think of standing up. My spinning head forced me right back on the floor. As the world turned and waves of nausea washed over me, feelings of guilt took hold. I wondered if I had missed the opportunity to head off this trouble before it spun out of control. I blamed myself for postponing the doctor's appointment upon our return. I blamed myself for not going to the hospital immediately after class.

My body felt limp. I was exhausted yet racked by anxiety. By now it was 1:00 a.m. Tuesday. My mind was racing with scores of questions for which I had no answers. What in the world had happened? I got flashbacks of diagrams depicting the anatomy of the ear.

I could not hear. This might be due to damage within the cochlea, the snail-shaped inner-ear organ that houses highly specialized hearing hair cells. We get a set number of those cells, and they must last us for a lifetime. Once dead or seriously damaged, they do not regenerate in humans. Instead, they are replaced by scar tissue. Of course, one of their biggest enemies is noise, and I'd had an excessively loud noise exposure at that church fund-raiser. I imagined that some of my hearing cells must have been beaten down by the sound waves, the way wheat stalks are flattened by strong winds in the fields.

Another scary thought that popped into my mind was the possibility that the cochlear nerve, or hearing nerve, might have sustained injury. This nerve relays electrical sound signals to the brain. If the nerve is dead, the patient is deaf. Although it is available, technology for helping people with non-functioning hearing nerves still needs perfecting. I also wondered if I might have had a "stroke of the ear." Any interruption or sudden decrease in blood flow to the very fine vessels that feed the ear can cause serious trouble immediately. It seemed plausible that a stress-induced spasm in a critical blood vessel might have something to do with my predicament. Stress narrows blood vessels, and the afternoon of the "event" had not been short of pressure and tension. But what if it was a blood clot? I did not even want to think about that option.

I could hardly lift my head, but my mind kept feeding me scenarios at a constant pace, like frames of an old home movie. Could a fluid buildup due to infection or inflammation have exerted enough pressure to choke the life out of my tiny ear structures? I had certainly had ample exposure to microbes of all kinds on the Alaskan trip. Plenty of humanity means plenty of germs. It was just my hunch, but if an infectious cause was a possibility, I put my money on the viral theory. I found out later that many patients who experience a sudden hearing loss report a recent viral infection.

It was certain that my balance system had taken a hit; hence, the nausea, the spinning sensations, the inability to stand up or walk. The sudden realization that my entire inner ear was involved brought on a panic attack. I will never forget being in the grip of such desperation and devastation. What a nightmare! It became clear that I needed help at once, with major efforts being directed toward damage control. Maybe there was still a way of stemming some of the destruction.

After what seemed like an eternity, the nausea and vomiting subsided a bit. Once again, my husband insisted that we had to go to the hospital—*now*. He threatened to call the ambulance. No, I told him, he could drive me. I crept on all fours to the stairs, sat on the top step, and gently eased myself down, one step at a time. Then, I crawled to the back door at a snail's pace. Keeping the body's center of gravity as low to the ground as possible sort of quelled the nausea. A slow-motion heave-ho from my husband got me into the car. It was now 2:00 a.m., Tuesday.

CHAPTER 4
In Search of Medical Help

A major medical center is located a short distance from our house. The ride there turned into a rather harrowing experience. I never realized that the street was in such bad shape. Every bump, every pothole, every turn made the world spin once again, like an out-of-control merry-go-round. I shut my eyes and pressed my hands against them. Any hint of light made the dizziness worse and brought a return of the dreaded nausea. It felt like we were breaking the sound barrier as the car "flew" down the road at a record-breaking speed of 20 miles per hour.

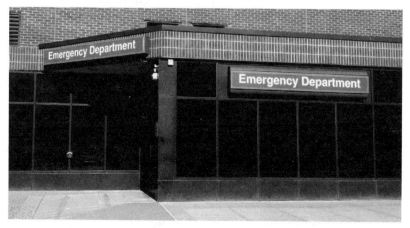

As the author learned, sudden hearing loss is a medical emergency.
photo: R.Hammond

When we finally arrived at the emergency room entrance, I stumbled through the doors, still hanging on to my bucket. Thankfully, it was only a short wait before I saw a doctor. He classified me as a patient with acute dehydration who needed IV (intravenous) fluids and a battery of blood tests. As soon as the needle was in my arm, I begged for medication. Shaking and in a clammy, cold sweat, I had rarely felt so poorly in my life. The heaves surged and waned but would not quit. At that point, I did not care anymore about the hearing loss. I just wanted to stop the world from spinning and bring the retching under control. The nurse finally gave me a dose of anti-nausea medicine. It was a good start, but I felt I needed more, a lot more; double or triple the dose, a whole quart maybe, whatever it would take to feel human again. Then, as the IV fluids and medications started to work, I had a fleeting light moment, punctuated by a giggle. For some reason I remembered a line from the 1973 Woody Allen movie, *Sleeper*: "At least after death you're not nauseous."

As the physician questioned and examined me, his very first impression was that I might be in the middle of a *benign paroxysmal positional vertigo* (BPPV) episode. BPPV is a common cause of dizziness. The doctor asked if I had sustained a recent head injury, if I had bent down too fast, or if I had tilted my head too far backward. No, I could not relate my dizziness to any particular event involving head movements of any kind.

In BPPV, the main players are little crystals called *otoconia,* or ear rocks. These are located within the balance system of the inner ear and are important for maintaining stability. If otoconia become loose and float outside of their assigned places, into areas where they do not belong, the patient becomes dizzy, nauseous, and unstable. Since the cochlea, or hearing organ, is not affected, however, this theory did not account for my hearing loss—and my left ear was totally deaf.

Another option was *vestibular neuritis.* This condition is believed to be due to a viral infection of the vestibular nerve, which leads from the balance structures of the inner ear to the brain. Again, patients become dizzy and ill, but they do not lose their hearing.

14

The doctor inquired if I'd had the flu or a cold prior to this event. No, except for some ear-thumping noises and maybe a slight transient queasiness, I had little to report. My symptoms actually matched the general description of a condition known as *viral labyrinthitis,* which typically affects all of the inner ear structures. It is usually caused by a virus and less often by bacteria. Symptoms, which can come on suddenly, include vertigo, dizziness, nausea, vomiting, imbalance, tinnitus (ringing in the ears), and some degree of hearing loss or hearing distortion. My being totally deaf in the left ear, however, was considered to be rather unusual.

As far as I recall, we never settled on a specific diagnosis during the emergency room visit. At 3:30 a.m., the nurse told me that I could go home as soon as the IV bag was empty, and she presented me with two prescription vials. One medication was for nausea control. The other one was intended to stabilize the confused inner-ear balance structures, which in turn would prevent further nausea. With plenty of rest, she assured me, I should improve within a few days. She did advise me, however, to consult my own physician as soon as possible.

Now I became a tad desperate. I did not feel like leaving without a reasonable explanation for my predicament. I needed at least some logical answers before I would get off the gurney. I explained, as calmly as possible, that the one-sided deafness both worried and frightened me. I did not want to go home and waste possibly precious time waiting for doctor appointments and maybe referrals. Obviously, something had gone terribly awry. Was there an ear specialist in the house? Unbeknownst to me, arrangements had already been made.

Around 4:00 a.m., the emergency doctor stepped into the room. While I was talking to the nurse, he had contacted the ENT (ear, nose, and throat) resident in the hospital. The order was to continue the hydration and nausea control. At 8:00 a.m. sharp, I was to come to the ENT clinic for hearing tests and a specialist consult. This was remarkable, as the average waiting period for a new patient to see a

15

doctor in that office was anywhere from three to six months.

This resident doctor evidently ran a tight ship and became my angel. I cannot describe what a relief it was to get a specialist's opinion on the issue. Had I left, I would have wondered for the rest of my life whether chances for improvement were squandered at a crucial moment. Maybe my ear would have repaired itself to its present point without help, but I am convinced that rapid medical intervention was beneficial. I stood my ground, and I have never regretted that decision.

CHAPTER 5
Interviews with the Specialists

At 8:00 a.m., I was sitting in a wheelchair in the waiting room of the ENT clinic. Hearing tests were first on the agenda. I had never had any of those assessments before. In fact, my hearing had always been my sharpest sense. When our pediatrician tested me as a child by means of the tuning fork, she could walk halfway across the room, and I still heard the vacillating *ying-ying* sounds.

Finally, a lady called my name, and so I met my first hearing science expert, the *audiologist*. She checked the insides of both ears. She asked what had happened but was not very keen on listening to too many details. Then she briefly explained the different tests that she would run and told me about my role in the process. I liked the part where the instruments recorded information, and I did not have to do anything. For this, the audiologist put some tightly fitting probes into the ears. I felt a slight pressure, and I could feel the eardrums pulsate. On my right ear I also heard some buzzing sounds, but that was pretty much it. This was easy enough.

The real test, however, was coming right up. I was led to a soundproof booth and had to sit on a chair. This time, the specialist inserted skinny earplug-like probes into the ears and handed me a clicker. Every time that I heard a beeping sound, no matter how faint, I had to push the button. Then she closed the rather impressive door.

First, the right ear was put through the steps. I figured that I identified that series of beeps in a satisfactory manner because we moved on to the left ear pretty quickly. I sat and waited. Nothing. Had she started the beeping yet? Then I detected a few very low-pitched *burr* sounds ... and then nothing. The door opened. Now the audiologist fitted me with a rather tight headband to which a coil was attached. The coil rested snuggly behind my left ear. Again, I had to listen for sounds. I thought that I heard a couple of very low-pitched signals. After a while, I felt a very faint vibration. The door swung open. We were done. I was close to tears.

I asked what the tests showed. The specialist was tight-lipped. She told me that the doctor liked to explain the results to new patients. When I insisted on a sneak preview, she did share that the left ear indeed recorded a loss. With that, I was wheeled back to the waiting room.

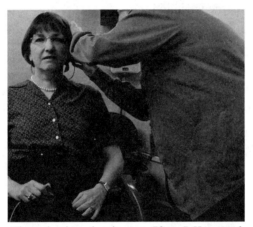

The author has a hearing test. *Photo R.Hammond*

I did not like hearing tests. Concentrating on those elusive beeps had been a very stressful experience that had given me a headache. By now, the medications that had been administered in the emergency room had reached their desired effect. I felt somewhat better, although I was terribly tired. I still did not know what was wrong with me, and I was ready to give up and go home ... but the day was still young.

Around 9:00 a.m., after the hearing tests, I met the *resident physician*, Dr. Todd. My spirits lifted; I liked Dr. Todd at once. I wondered if he had run interference for me in the wee hours of the morning and short-circuited that insane waiting period, but I did not ask.

Dr. Todd was a very professional, no-nonsense young man, and for a while I even thought that he might be *the* specialist whom I had been sent to see. He was well informed about the details of my disturbing incident, and he had a plan for how and where to search for a possible explanation. He inspected my ears once more but did not find anything abnormal. He sat down and studied the hearing test report, or audiogram. He agreed that I had a profound left-sided hearing loss. The tests for the right ear looked normal. Then he performed a neurological exam. He made me follow his finger with my eyes. Zoom! Zoom! Look here, there, everywhere. Although my eyes watered at once, I thought that I did well tracking the roving index finger. Then I found out that I tested seriously positive for nystagmus, or involuntary, rhythmic, rapid eye movements. Considering my condition, Dr. Todd was not amazed. He felt that my eye jerks were related to abnormal activity in the inner-ear balance system, or vestibular system. He mentioned the need for an MRI scan. It would look for general damage to the ear structures, bone injuries, and fluid leakage. Mostly, it would search for tumors—of the brain, in general, and of the hearing and balance nerves, specifically.

Even though the doctor remained cautiously optimistic that the scan would be fine, I began to lose it emotionally. He tried to curb my already heightened state of anxiety by telling me that in cases like mine, an MRI was a routine procedure. I knew that the word "tumor" simply means a swelling, a mass, or a growth. It does not necessarily imply cancer or malignancy. Yet deep down in my gut, that is what I was afraid of. I began to worry about all sorts of unsettling scenarios.

Speaking in an encouraging tone, Dr. Todd gave me an A+ for

coming in early. I wondered about a diagnosis, but we had only just begun the testing. He did have a hunch, he said, yet he could not share it until the specialist, his boss, had given his opinion. A firm diagnosis might be weeks away. He mentioned that it can be hard to sort out the often-conflicting findings and test results until the body has found its cadence again and has done some healing. The doctors would do their best to prevent further injury, if at all possible. He reassured me that I had gotten lucky because the specialist that I was about to see was the best. What a lovely thing to say about his mentor.

Dr. Todd continued to ask scores of questions and took lengthy notes. Relevant information that guides the doctor toward a diagnosis is often hidden in the details of the patient's health history and account of events. Together, we reviewed the already cited conditions that might have led to symptoms similar to mine. Barring any new discoveries, we came up with the theory that made the most sense— the theory of the "perfect ear storm." Three unrelated events—a possible viral infection, excessive noise exposure, and a high-stress situation—might very well have contributed to my hearing loss and balance issues. Too much, it seemed, had happened at once.

To my relief, Dr. Todd said that after all the tests were done, I would get some medications that he felt could be helpful. He did not extend promises of a cure or even improvement, but he hoped that the medicines would stem further damage and support my ear during the healing process. He warned me that I would need patience, which is not my best trait. If I regained any hearing, it would probably happen within the first few weeks, but it might not be "useful" hearing, at least not at the outset. It might improve a bit and refine itself, but there were no guarantees. I should expect that my hearing would never be the same.

I did not realize it at the time, but I had just embarked on a journey of discovery that would teach me a lot about myself and about what medicine can and cannot do. My new life had just begun in earnest.

A little before 10:00 a.m., the *ENT specialist,* Dr. Leonard, joined us. As he grabbed the audiogram, I told him that I knew about my rather steep left hearing loss. "You are deaf in the ear" was his response. I guess there was no need to gloss over the obvious, but it was tough to hear it said out loud. Dr. Leonard reviewed Dr. Todd's notes and asked him a few questions. He also redid the nystagmus assessment; he wanted to see for himself, he said. Then the doctors set out to make me walk a straight line in order to test my balance. This struck me as a bit amusing, as I could hardly sit in the chair without listing. Assisted by my husband, they got me on my feet. I took a couple of very wobbly steps and crashed against the wall. Both physicians grabbed me just in time before I fell down, face first. What a helpless feeling it was to keel over without having any control whatsoever in catching myself. Dr. Todd was most concerned about my being a serious fall risk. Yet he tried to convince me not to get too upset. The balance would improve with time. There were things that I could do to help myself.

Both doctors reminded me, however, that taking a tumble and breaking a hip was not in my best interest. The nurse would give me instruction sheets for specific equilibrium exercises, if my husband promised not to let me practice unattended. In addition, in case that I was unable to manage, I could be referred to a therapist for special classes devoted entirely to balance retraining. Dr. Todd pepped me up by reminding me how miraculously the body and the brain can adjust to changes. I have thought a lot about his wise statement over the years.

Finally, Dr. Leonard sat down and gave me his opinion. He supported the "perfect ear storm" theory, but he said we still had loads of unknowns. He mentioned that there were many more reasons why people lose their hearing. He pelted me with questions that involved my own health history and that of my family. He was also most curious about our ear and hearing histories. He wanted to know if I was aware of any autoimmune disorders, such as lupus, among my blood relatives. He covered ear surgeries, ear infections, childhood diseases, medications and supplements, head trauma, noise levels at home and at work, and more. The thought of an autoimmune component worried me. I was reassured that until we knew more, I would be given medication to cover some of the possible causes for a sudden hearing loss such as mine. The corticosteroid prednisone (e.g. *Deltasone, Orasone*) would work on inflammation and immunity concerns. I answered all of the questions as best I could, although the reason for asking some of them escaped me at that time.

Suddenly, there was a knock at the door. The results for some of the blood tests that had been drawn earlier in the ER were back. The physicians huddled around the computer and then stepped into the hall. I never got all the details, but quite a few of the blood chemistry reports were abnormal. Dr. Leonard decided to admit me to the hospital for electrolyte corrections, a whole battery of additional blood tests, further nausea management, the start of a medication program, and, of course, the administration of an MRI exam.

CHAPTER 6
The Hospital Stay

By 1:00 p.m., I was in my shared room on the neurology floor. If I had thought I would have a moment of peace, I was wrong. I had a high-maintenance roommate. Visitors streamed in and out, and someone brought in containers of highly fragrant foods. That was all I needed. Once again, I became violently ill.

Luckily, I met yet another angel, Nurse Lisa. She was very calm and comforting. She summoned the IV specialist at once so that a new line would be started for continued hydration fluids. She mentioned that she was anxious to give me another dose of anti-nausea medication. In a firm yet diplomatic way, Lisa convinced my neighbor's family to remove the smelly leftovers. Then she posted a big sign on the door and by my bed, warning that I was on "fall precautions": under no circumstance was I to get up by myself. The lab tech stopped by and drew more blood.

By mid-afternoon, I felt a bit better. Nurse Lisa helped me change into a hospital gown in preparation for the MRI scan. I had to surrender any jewelry and was quizzed about other metal materials, such as hairpins or safety pins that might be attracted by the MRI machine's magnets. As serious harm could be caused due to internal metal parts and batteries, I was cautioned that materials and devices such as a pacemaker, an ear implant, a hip or knee prosthesis, pumps, or stents would need the approval of the radiologist before the test could be performed. "Any metals with magnetic properties will be sucked right up," Nurse Lisa warned. For afternoon snack, I got a hefty antiviral pill. Since the retching had subsided, Nurse Lisa tried to coax me into also taking my first dose of prednisone. Having dispensed loads of this drug during my long pharmacy career, I knew that it has a reputation for causing serious stomach upsets. I had not eaten a thing and worried that I might get sick during the test, which could compromise the hugely expensive scanner. Finally, Lisa's persistence paid off. I gave in and swallowed the tablet. The MRI was scheduled for around 4:00 p.m.

Before I knew it, the orderly arrived, and three people helped me onto the cart. Nurse Lisa warned the transporter to be a gentle driver. She leaned over and whispered into my good ear that by the time I got back, she would have taken care of the roommate situation. She had her eye on a private room where I might get some rest. This came as great news; things were finally looking up. Then Lisa tucked a small basin under the blanket, and we were off.

We started out easily, but as the orderly's pager kept buzzing, we picked up speed. We raced down the hall and zoomed around one corner and then another. A quick 90-degree turn landed us in the elevator. *Ding, ding*—we stopped on every floor. Again, my stomach began to turn. Then, with a *clunk-clunk,* the cart jerked out of the elevator, and we headed down a seemingly endless hall. As the ceiling lights swept by above my head, the world went into a spin. I felt around for the basin, pinched my eyes shut, and tried to pull the cover over my head. Might we slow down a bit? No worries, the orderly assured me; we were almost there. Around two more sharp corners and—stop. We had arrived. The wild ride taught me that I had never appreciated the great job that my inner ears do for keeping me steady, even under the most challenging of circumstances.

The MRI tech greeted us. He wanted me to "hop off" the gurney and onto the scanner table. I asked for a minute of reprieve to collect myself before I moved. I had to let the dizziness subside. Then I sat up very carefully, pressed my clammy hands against my eyes, and took some slow, deep breaths. It was cold in the room.

While I tried to get my bearings, the tech fired off a few questions.

He wondered if I had any metal on me or in me. No, Nurse Lisa had taken care of that. When I mentioned that I was somewhat claustrophobic, he wanted to know if the nurse had given me any sedation medication. She had not. He suggested that I might want to listen to some music, and an assistant gave me a set of earphones. I was told that the test would take about thirty-five minutes, and I felt that I could manage that. The technician also mentioned that the "tube" was equipped with an audio system that was in operation during the scan. All I had to do was talk, and he would hear me in the control room. I was given an emergency clicker. A push of the panic button would stop the test immediately. I reclined ever so slowly onto the table. I remember that my head was positioned into some type of contraption and then I was guided into the scanner. It was a tight fit.

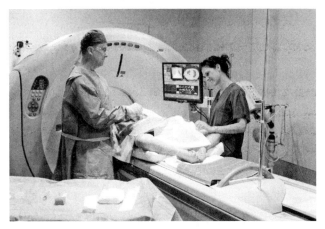

Instructions are given before an MRI Scan.
photo: (c) epstock www.fotosearch.com

I knew the MRI tube could induce anxiety reactions in claustrophobic people. As a pharmacist, I had dispensed plenty of medications meant to keep patients comfortable during the test. What I did *not* know was how terribly loud the machine would be. I closed

25

my eyes, yet I could not resist a peek. Almost at eyebrow level was a mirror that showed the inside of the room I was in. The tech's console was off to the right. This optical illusion assured me that I was not encased like a mummy and alone. Anyway, it helped as I tried to relax.

Relax? *Brrr, brrr, bam, bam.* It sounded as if a pile driver was at work right next to my head. I was not prepared for this and began to worry about my right ear. The headphones did not fit tightly enough and were of little help. Trusting that the audio was on, I called out, "Hello! This is dangerously loud."

"That's the nature of the beast," a voice came back over the intercom. In the end, I did survive the MRI scan, and the orderly brought me back to the nursing station.

***

Nurse Lisa had gotten me a very nice private room. Unfortunately, I couldn't sleep. I was antsy and worried. I heard funny noises, almost like garbled voices, in my left ear. Off and on, a most annoying buzz or hiss would break through. Also, it seemed that every five minutes, medical staff came to check on something. Whenever I wanted to get up, I had to call for help. I tried to watch TV, but I could not concentrate. Wednesday morning came slowly.

When breakfast time finally arrived, it also was time for more pills. By mid-morning, my blood pressure was up, and I felt mighty jittery and restless—that was bad. I suspected the culprit was the prednisone. Steroidal anti-inflammatories are notorious for causing salt and water retention and for revving up energy levels.

By the time Dr. Todd came to visit, however, I had some good news to share. On my pillow speaker, I could hear faint voices. Without looking at the TV, I was able to tell if a man or a woman was talking. I could not understand a word of their conversation, but Dr. Todd was not concerned. He gave this new development a very positive rating. Sound signals were getting through to the brain. We would hold a good thought, take anything we got, and hope for more.

Dr. Todd also had good news for me. The MRI did not show any tumors or other miscellaneous damage. I told him about my ear-shattering scanner experience. He guessed that I might have acquired some *hyperacusis*, a condition when everything seems way too loud. That could exaggerate an already bad situation. In time, it might settle down. When I asked about the "ear noises," he became more pensive. He feared that I was coming down with *tinnitus*, commonly referred to as "ringing in the ears." It might go away, but considering the seriousness of the hearing loss, it might not. The latter turned out to be true.

***

After a short debate, my physician tag team decided to keep me in the hospital for another day. Besides my blood pressure issue, my balance had not improved to where it was safe to discharge me. Hanging on to the IV pole, I shuffled around the room as my attendant coached me: "Hold your head up straight. Don't stoop. Don't look at your feet. Focus on an object and walk toward it."

Gradually, I gained a bit of confidence and walked on my own—well, somewhat. My blood pressure, however, kept rising, and the heart rate followed suit. The nurse called the doctor. Shortly thereafter, Dr. Leonard showed up, dressed in his surgical scrubs. He also bet that the prednisone was at fault, yet he was amazed that I had such a phenomenal reaction after taking just a few tablets. He ordered a lower dose and started me on *Dyazide*, a combination of two drugs used to treat fluid retention. Getting rid of some extra water would help manage the creeping pressure. It was a good thing that the "fall precautions" had been lifted. Otherwise, I would have been on that call button all afternoon and night as I needed numerous trips to the bathroom. Wobbling back and forth between the bed and the facilities, my balance system got a workout. Earlier, the nurse had pulled the IV and convinced me to try a diet of bland, solid foods. Except for feeling like a bloated, frenzied balloon with an out-of-control cardiovascular system, I was doing better.

***

During my hospital stay, a lot of different tests were done. When I wondered why, Dr. Todd told me that hearing loss, as well as dizziness and balance problems, are often not related directly to the ear itself. Instead, they can be symptoms of other underlying conditions. Although tests might not answer all the questions, they help the physician when deciding on a diagnosis or further medical investigations.

Throughout the book, I will recall these important points in the appropriate sections. They reinforce the fact that people with hearing and ear-related complaints would do well to consult a doctor who specializes in ear disorders. With test data on hand, the physician will be able to weigh the options and suggest an action plan.

CHAPTER 7
Going Home

On Thursday morning a different doctor came to visit; he was filling in for Dr. Leonard. He announced that I was ready to go home and wrote a bunch of prescriptions. The prednisone was meant to decrease any inflammation in my ear and to cool down a possibly excited immune system. It was to continue for a total of a month, which did not come as a surprise. After two weeks of high-dose treatment, the gradual tapering-off schedule would begin. The physician gave me the standard warning—stopping this medication abruptly, or "cold turkey," could very well lead to another ER visit. During my years of pharmacy practice, I witnessed the consequences of such action many times and did not plan on putting myself unnecessarily at risk.

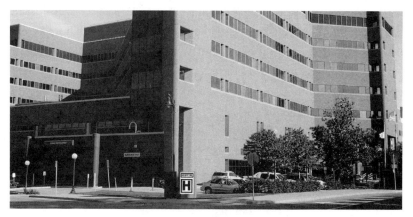

The author is discharged from the Hospital. *photo: R.Hammond*

Since the blood pressure did not want to relent, we would definitely continue the *Dyazide* for fluid and blood pressure management. The

29

next prescription was for the stomach acid-reducer ranitidine (*Zantac*). It would deal with the digestive upset that prednisone frequently causes, especially at high doses. The doctor kept writing. Just in case a virus had invaded my ear and/or its nerves, I needed to complete the full ten-day course of the antiviral medication. It would keep the virus from multiplying, which would hopefully stop the damage. Once the culprit was immobilized, chances were good that the immune system would "neutralize" it. This sounded almost like warfare, and I guess it was. The doctor mentioned that I might regain some hearing, but only time would tell how much harm had already been done—that was in agreement with what Dr. Todd had already told me.

Next, he prescribed low-dose diazepam (*Valium*), as it was expected to do a good job in calming my overly active, confused inner ear balance system. Also, its anxiety-blunting effect would make it easier to deal with the tinnitus that by now had become truly annoying. I hoped that it might also grant me a few hours of sleep.

I asked the discharge physician about my diagnosis. Truthfully, I was a bit afraid of the answer. Over the last two days, we had discussed many potential causes for my predicament, some of which unsettled me. I was told that for now—and that might still change—I had left-sided *sudden sensorineural hearing loss* (SSHL). Dr. Leonard would discuss the details and any unresolved issues later. I wondered what could change the diagnosis. The answer was that we would have to wait and see if my episode marked the beginning of *Ménière's disease,* a disorder of the inner ear that affects both hearing and balance. For now, all options had to remain on the table. Obviously, the tests had not revealed any answers yet, which was disappointing, but I did not feel like asking for further details.

Finally, I was cautioned to limit salt intake, relax, manage my stress, and get plenty of rest. Within three weeks, I was to return for another hearing check, followed by an appointment with Dr. Leonard. The doctor started to leave but then stopped to admonish me: until that time, no driving was allowed.

As the door closed, a sense of utter hopelessness overcame me. Suddenly, it seemed that there were more problems than answers. The magnitude and possible ramifications of the situation totally overwhelmed me. I wondered what the future would hold. Would I ever be able to work again? I had trouble understanding speech in noise, and the tinnitus wore me out. How would all of this impact my life? What if the vertigo came back? Nobody had even ventured a guess on these issues. Time would tell.

I fumbled around the room and, hanging on to the walls and bed, I gathered my belongings. I wanted to say good-bye to Nurse Lisa, but she was not scheduled to work, and I never saw her again. The same was true for Dr. Todd.

I sat in the chair and waited for Ross to pick me up. The nurse on duty offered a last blood pressure check, but I did not care anymore about the numbers and refused. I was ready to leave.

CHAPTER 8
New Realities

I walked—or more like weaved—into the house under my own power. I decided to camp out in the den until I knew whether I would be able to sleep at night. That way, I could watch TV and maybe read without keeping my husband up all night. It turned out to be a good decision. The doctor's instructions to relax and rest were incompatible with the prednisone, which does have the reputation for pepping people up. Never before did I have the urge to wash the kitchen floor at three in the morning or to clean the attic and the oven all at the same time. Between my buzzing ear and my jittery brain, I simply could not figure out how to unwind. The suggestion that I should "take it easy" turned into wishful thinking.

As time went on, many of my initial hopes were dashed. I had hoped that the stuffy feeling would clear out of my ear. I had hoped that the tinnitus might loosen its grip. Sometimes, in the early morning hours, I thought that it had let up a bit—but before long, it would kick back into high gear. Every day Ross took me for a short walk in the neighborhood. It did not take much to throw me off kilter—kids playing on the sidewalk, planes overhead, cars coming toward us. The world had become excessively loud and bright. Pretty soon, I could not be outside without wearing sunglasses. As my balance was challenged, my eyes began to water. I kept wandering off into the bushes and tripped over just about anything. Walking had become a hazardous activity. When I rode in the car, I could barely stand the droning road noise. Going grocery shopping became a torture. I could hardly hear, yet I had to turn the TV volume down. Was this going to be my life? As I neared my three-week recheck appointment, I wrote down some of my observations and a number of questions for Dr. Leonard.

***

During my follow-up visit, the hearing tests took a bit longer. My left ear indeed showed some improvement. I recorded enough beeps for the audiologist to add a *word recognition* test. It consisted of a series of spoken, one-syllable words that I had to repeat correctly. My score was an impressive 28 percent, which totally amazed Dr. Leonard. I had regained a lot more hearing than he had thought possible. He kept my diagnosis as sudden sensorineural hearing loss (SSNL) and expressed the hope that I would make more progress.

I finally inquired about *Ménière's disease*. The discharge physician had left that option open, and I wondered if I had it. Dr. Leonard did not think that I was a Ménière's patient, although my violent vertigo attack was reminiscent of this condition. Still, there were few ways of telling for sure. My question regarding the need for further testing did not bring on a wave of enthusiasm. I learned that there were no definitive tests for diagnosing Ménière's disease. I had already had the initial evaluations, such as a physical checkup, an MRI, diagnostic hearing tests, and blood screens that are commonly performed on people suspected of the disorder. So far, there were no particular red flags; only time would tell. Because I was holding my own and improving, he did not see any reason to put me through more tests at this point. However, if I should I come down with episodes similar to the one that I had just experienced, we would have to dig deeper. For the time being, he told me, I had plenty to get used to, and so we would leave things as they were.

I had yet another question. I wondered why everything was so loud. The doctor admitted that this was hard to explain. The production of an overly intense, substandard sound signal was the direct result of my sudden, profound hearing loss. The sound sensing and processing capabilities of the cochlea were severely challenged due to dead

34

and damaged hearing cells. Besides, possible nerve damage could also contribute to the annoyance. However, there was a chance for improvement with time. My ear had taken a major hit, and we might never know what happened or why. Dr. Leonard cautioned me to be mindful of loud noise but not to overprotect my ears with tight earplugs and the like. He acknowledged that this was a delicate balancing act and felt that it would be wise to discuss proper ear protection strategies with the audiologist.

***

In the beginning I tried hard to keep life as normal as possible. Although it had not yet registered with me, the "old normal" was gone. Two weeks after the event, I went back to teaching. I finished the fifteen-week cycle that I had started and promptly signed up for another semester, although I wonder now what I was thinking. Within a month, I was back at my hospital job. Everybody thought that I coped really well, but it soon became obvious that I had to cut back on my shifts. I had trouble understanding conversation over the din in the pharmacy. What was that patient's allergy? Lasix or latex? Noise and stress drove my tinnitus into orbit. It literally took me longer to "hear." I had trouble locating noise sources, such as ringing telephones and beeping pagers, and my balance issues only added to the problem. I spent a tremendous amount of energy trying to keep up with full work days while running on half-power. I was introduced to the notions of "listening fatigue" and "listening effort" that so challenge those with hearing loss. Although I tried my best, it was increasingly hard to function safely and effectively in the noise-confused place that the pharmacy had become. Eventually, the realization that life had changed forever took me out of my "normal" environment and pointed me in a new direction and toward new opportunities and a new life mission. And that was good.

Chapter 9
Moving On

Three months after the ear event, I had yet another visit with Dr. Leonard. At this point, the hearing test results remained basically unchanged. This meant that the hearing loss had stabilized. It looked like further improvement in my problem hearing ranges could no longer be expected. Both the doctor and the audiologist, however, were almost awed by my 72 percent word recognition test score, which suggested that my understanding of speech had improved. Unfortunately, in real life this did not hold true. Normal conversations do not consist of one-syllable words and do not take place in soundproof booths.

Doctor Leonard released me from acute care and suggested that I might explore the option of a hearing aid. I did not know much about hearing assistance in general, so I asked all sorts of questions. This is when I found out that physicians are not very well versed on hearing aids. Dr. Leonard recommended that I schedule a meeting with a clinic audiologist for a hearing aid evaluation and introductory class. This turned out to be very good advice.

Roughly six months after the incident, I also started to attend support group meetings, and I still do. Although they are not helpful for everyone, for me it is time well spent. I feel that it is hard to face the fallout of life-changing events all alone. Besides, it is remarkable how much one can learn from peers. Meeting other people and hearing about their issues and challenges shined a totally new light on my own problems.

Overall, it took about a year before I accepted my hearing loss and its accompanying side effects as part of my life. It was not an easy road—one that was fraught with frustration, anger, regret, and a lot of work. The best treatment that I got for myself was to learn about the condition, from all angles, until the pieces of the puzzle that is hearing loss gradually fell into place. In so many ways, education turned out to be both liberating and empowering. It did not change anything, but it steered me toward some amazing discoveries that had been concealed under a cloak of pain and trauma. The time had come to accept the "new me" and to move on.

PART TWO
A JOURNEY of DISCOVERY

Chapter 10
Steep Learning Curve

In pharmacy college, I studied the anatomy and function of the ear quite extensively, including an introduction to the basic elements of the physics of sound. As expected, most of the courses concentrated on drug therapies, which included those for different ear disorders, particularly infections. I learned how to dose and monitor patients who were treated with ototoxic, or ear-harmful, medications. Although I used the expressions such as tinnitus and vertigo regularly, I never knew what they felt like. On the night when rather abstract medical concepts suddenly turned into my reality, I discovered that the ears still held plenty of mysteries. They had never been the primary focus of my practice, and now I found out that many conditions, like hearing loss itself, tinnitus, recruitment, hyperacusis, and Ménière's disease, lay outside of my comfort zone. There was a lot to learn. I was introduced overnight to audiology and hearing testing to which I had no previous personal or professional exposure. It was frustrating not to understand what my hearing test results meant. It took a while to realize it, but in order to deal with my situation I had to familiarize myself with the science behind the many challenges that suddenly affected me in a most personal way.

I was a diligent student. I wrote down my questions and concerns and took a notebook to all my appointments. Yet the answers that professionals gave me were often vague and uninformative. The different pieces of what seemed to be a gigantic puzzle did not come together. I assumed part of the blame for my confusion because I knew few specific details regarding the different ear and hearing issues that confronted me. Obviously, the learning curve was steep. As I set out on my fact-finding mission, I ran into some tough study material.

Along the way, I came to appreciate once more the wonders and complexities of the hearing and balance organs—the ears. To this day they hold many secrets, even for scientists, a fact that explained the rather hesitant explanations that my health care specialists frequently offered.

Chapter 11
Road Map for the Journey –
How the Ear Works

Before setting out on my journey into the world of hearing loss, I had to establish a reliable road map that would serve as my guide. Although it might be rather clinical in nature, I felt that a review of the most important features of the ear was a logical and necessary starting point. I had to fill in my knowledge gaps with those details and expressions that would facilitate my communicating with the professionals who cared for me. It might not seem like it, but what follows is a very basic description of the structures that help us hear and maintain our balance. It is easy to see how things can go wrong somewhere along the way. For me, it became essential to sort out these details in order to make any sense whatsoever of my case.

How the Ear Works: Anatomy and Function

The greatly simplified diagrams are for illustration purposes only. They are not drawn to scale. Some anatomic features are omitted and the perspective has been manipulated to show the approximate location of the hearing and balance structures discussed in this text.

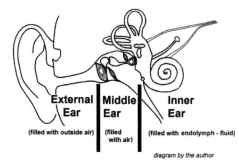

diagram by the author

43

The ear has three parts: the external ear, the middle ear, and the inner ear. The external and middle ear sections are exclusively involved with hearing. The inner ear has two functions; namely, hearing and balance.

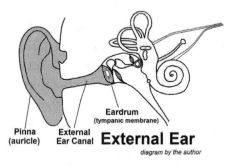

Eardrum
(tympanic membrane)

Pinna
(auricle)

External
Ear Canal **External Ear**

diagram by the author

The ***external ear*** consists of the *pinna*, or auricle, which is the visible portion of the ear, and of the *external ear canal*. The ear canal is a little over an inch long. It extends from the outside ear opening to the eardrum, or tympanic membrane. It is lined with fine hairs and special *glands* that secrete *cerumen,* which forms a lubricant and protectant barrier. Cerumen has a waxy consistency and is commonly called earwax. Too much cerumen impedes the free flow of sound waves through the ear canal, which can lead to decreased hearing and maybe even tinnitus, or noises in the ears.

The external ear captures airborne sound waves and funnels them through the ear canal to the tympanic membrane, which marks the transition between the outer and the middle ear. The sound waves hit the eardrum and cause it to vibrate.

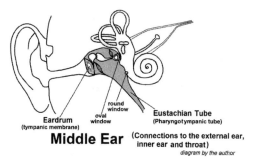

round
window
oval
Eardrum window
(tympanic membrane)

Eustachian Tube
(Pharyngotympanic tube)

Middle Ear (Connections to the external ear,
inner ear and throat)

diagram by the author

The *middle ear* is an air-filled chamber. It begins at the eardrum, which transforms sound waves into mechanical energy, or vibrations. The middle ear connects to the inner ear by means of two small, membrane-covered openings, which are referred to as "windows." They perforate the bone that separates the middle and the inner ear. Located one above the other, the upper window is known as the *oval window*, the lower one as the *round window*. The *eustachian tube* equalizes the air pressure on both sides of the eardrum. If the pressure across the eardrum is not equalized, the membrane cannot vibrate properly, which affects sound quality and intensity. The eustachian tube also links the middle ear to the throat, or pharynx, and acts as a drain pipe. Medical references often refer to it as the "pharyngotympanic tube."

45

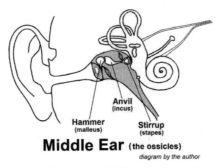

Middle Ear (the ossicles)
diagram by the author

The main players in the middle ear are three interconnected bones, the *ossicles,* which relay the vibrations from the eardrum to the inner ear.

The ossicles are the smallest bones in the body and are named mostly for their physical appearance. Starting at the eardrum, they are the *malleus*, or hammer, which attaches to the eardrum; the *incus*, or anvil; and the *stapes*, or stirrup, whose footplate fills the oval window. The ossicles form a chain of mechanical levers that act as a vibration relay and amplification system. Eardrum vibrations set the middle-ear ossicle chain into motion, starting at the malleus, progressing to the incus, and ending at the stapes, which communicates with the oval window, its connection to the inner ear.

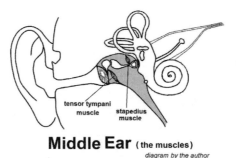

Middle Ear (the muscles)
diagram by the author

The middle ear also has two very tiny *muscles:* the *tensor tympani* attaches to the malleus, and the *stapedius muscle* attaches to the stapes. The exact purpose of these muscles is still unclear. They are said to have a stabilizing effect on the ossicle chain, and appear to harmonize, or modulate, sound vibrations. They shield the inner ear from excess noise by contracting when they are exposed to loud sound. Such muscle activity stiffens the eardrum and ossicle chain, which limits vibration transmission to the cochlea. The stapedius muscle is dominant in this protective function. Its reflex-type contraction is commonly measured during hearing tests as an indicator of middle ear function. Yet every reflex involves a *delay* between action and reaction, which raises the question to what extent stapedius contractions can insulate the inner ear from damage due to *sudden* loud noise insults.

The ***inner ear*** is involved with both hearing and balance, which will be addressed separately. But first, let's take a look at the inner ear as a whole.

Referred to as the "labyrinth"—which means maze—the inner ear has a complicated anatomy. The labyrinth is made of the *bony labyrinth*, which houses the *membranous labyrinth*.

47

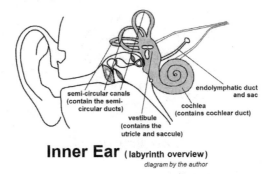

Inner Ear (labyrinth overview)

diagram by the author

The *bony labyrinth* consists of a series of hollow cavities and canals that are carved into the temporal bone of the skull. These are the cochlea, which is dedicated to hearing, and the vestibule and the semicircular canals, which are involved with balance. The cavities and canals of the bony labyrinth support and protect a series of interconnected *ducts* and *organs* collectively known as the *membranous labyrinth.* The major structures of the membranous labyrinth are the cochlear duct, two organs known as the utricle and saccule, the endolymphatic duct with the endolymphatic sac, and the semicircular ducts.

The spiral-shaped, bony cochlea holds the *cochlear duct.* The cavity of the vestibule, which lies roughly between the cochlea and the semicircular canals, shelters the *utricle* and the *saccule.* The three semicircular canals are lined with the *semicircular ducts.* Arising from the vestibular area is the *endolymphatic duct,* which is topped by the *endolymphatic sac.* This structure is protected by surrounding bone. It is thought to help regulate fluid pressure within the inner ear. The sac has also been found to have a defensive function and to play a role in the disposal of waste products and debris.

The membranous labyrinth is filled with a fluid called *endolymph.* It is surrounded by another fluid called *perilymph.* Those two liquids are confined to their own spaces and do not come into direct contact with one another.

The Inner Ear and Hearing

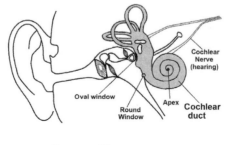

Inner Ear (hearing)
diagram by the author

The cochlear duct is a membranous tube that is filled with endolymph and coils like a snail, following the outline of its bony protective capsule. Inside are roughly 20,000 specialized *hair cells* that are often referred to as hearing cells. The hair cells are topped with very fine extensions, called *cilia*. Just as fibers are knotted into a carpet base, the hair cells are anchored in a membrane known as the basilar membrane. They are finely tuned to respond to all the various sound frequencies, or pitches, and volumes. Their signals are relayed to the brain by the *cochlear nerve*.

As the "snail" curls from the outside to its innermost point, or *apex*, the cells that are in charge of the high frequencies are located toward the entrance of the structure. They are followed by the mid-range frequency responders. Those that are tuned to the low frequencies are found toward the innermost curl of the snail. This tuned "hair cell coil" inside the cochlear duct is the actual *hearing organ*, which is known as the *organ of Corti*. We are born with a set number of these miraculous, fragile hair cells. They are extremely sensitive to injury, especially injury due to loud noise exposures. Once they are damaged or dead, they do not regenerate. Irreversible hearing loss and deafness are the obvious results.

Vibrations from the middle ear ossicles are transmitted to the inner ear by the stapes via the oval window. These vibrations ultimately cause endolymph movements within the cochlear duct that sway and bend the cilia. Responding to the motions of the cilia, the supporting hair cells translate the endolymph fluid action into electrical signals. By expanding and contracting, the membrane filling the *round window* serves as a relief valve equalizing pressure changes caused by the moving endolymph.

The Way to the Brain
The cochlear nerve carries the electrical messages generated by the cochlear hair cells to the brainstem. From here, the impulses are passed on upward to the hearing portion of the brain, or *auditory cortex,* for *processing, deciphering, and interpretation.* The way to the auditory cortex consists of an elaborate network of nerve fibers, complete with relay and switching points. In essence, we "hear" with our brain. We can have the most perfect ear structures ever, but if the nerve and brain connections do not function properly, we will not hear a thing—or what we hear might not make any sense.

The pathway of sound in ten steps

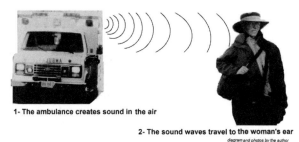

1- The ambulance creates sound in the air

2- The sound waves travel to the woman's ear
diagram and photos by the author

3- Sound waves enter the ear canal
and vibrate the eardrum
diagram by the author

4- Eardrum vibrations set middle ear
ossicles in motion
diagram by the author

5- The stapes vibrates the oval window

6- These vibrations produce wave movements
in the endolymph liquid of the inner ear
diagram by the author

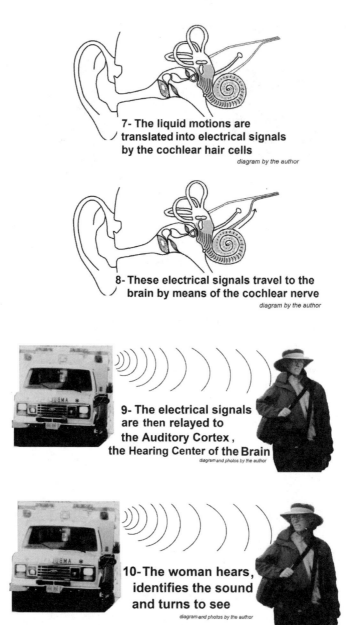

7- The liquid motions are translated into electrical signals by the cochlear hair cells

diagram by the author

8- These electrical signals travel to the brain by means of the cochlear nerve

diagram by the author

9- The electrical signals are then relayed to the Auditory Cortex , the Hearing Center of the Brain

diagram and photos by the author

10- The woman hears, identifies the sound and turns to see

diagram and photos by the author

The Inner Ear and Balance

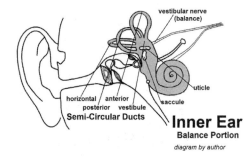

Inner Ear
Balance Portion
diagram by author

A separate function of the inner ear is that it helps us maintain our equilibrium. This is the job of the specialized cells of the *three semicircular ducts* and of the *utricle* and *saccule*, which are referred to as the *"otoliths,"* or "ear stone" organs. Together, these five structures are known as the *vestibular system* or *vestibular apparatus*. Their connection to the brain is the *vestibular nerve*.

The semicircular ducts contain motion sensor cells that monitor head movements in three directions: anterior, posterior, and horizontal. The otoliths organs help us keep our balance, especially in response to gravity.

Whether we are on the go or at rest, the inner-ear balance/equilibrium systems provide the brain with information about body motion as well as head movements and positions. They also maintain nervous connections to the eyes and to special receptor cells located in muscles, joints, and tendons. It takes the teamwork of all three systems—inner ears, eyes, and body sensors—to keep us from falling, even under the most adverse conditions.

The Eighth Cranial Nerve

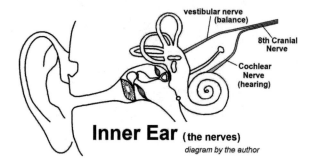

Inner Ear (the nerves)
diagram by the author

As noted earlier, the cochlear cells send their electrical signals to the brain by means of the cochlear nerve, while the vestibular system communicates with designated brain areas via the vestibular nerve. Together, these two nerve trunks make up the *vestibulo-cochlear* nerve, also known as the *eighth cranial nerve*. The branches are wrapped and insulated by special cells called *Schwann cells*.

Chapter 12
Audiology and Hearing Tests

As I found out on the morning after my ear event, the obvious first stop for people with hearing loss is the audiologist's office. I was told that I needed a comprehensive set of hearing tests before I could see the specialist. Although my hearing had never been formally tested before, I understood that the purpose of the session was to determine how much I heard on each ear and to document any hearing loss. I did not know what types of assessments would be done or how they would be done. I also did not know their diagnostic value or how they could explain what ailed me.

Audiology is the science of hearing, a complex topic tied intimately to physics and math. The lady who performed my hearing evaluation was an *audiologist*, or hearing specialist. When the testing was over, I received a report, called an *audiogram,* to bring to my doctor. Although multiple hearing tests were eventually done, I never received a satisfactory explanation of what the results revealed about my hearing loss or how the findings would influence treatment choices. Had I known more about audiology, I would have been able to ask concise questions.

It has taken me a while to figure out which assessments are commonly performed in order to diagnose a patient's type and extent of hearing loss. I have learned the hard way that hearing-challenged people need a basic understanding of the different tests so they can open a meaningful dialogue with their specialists. I have also learned that I should always ask for a copy of my audiograms. This information is very helpful in case I should need to go elsewhere for medical care or for a hearing aid consult.

Testing the Whole Ear

On the morning of my first audiology appointment, the audiologist told me that the first series of hearing assessments is usually the most comprehensive. The challenge is to get a feeling for the type, location, and severity of the hearing loss. A whole litany of tests is used to evaluate different areas and functions of the ear. The audiologist determines the combinations and types of evaluations that will be administered on a case-by-case basis, as every hearing loss is different. Some tests are now standard for me, while others are not done because I do not need them or they are not helpful.

At the start of my first testing session, the specialist informed me that each ear would be evaluated separately. We would start with the outer structure, the pinna, move along the ear canal, and work our way to the sanctum of hearing, the cochlear cells of the inner ear.

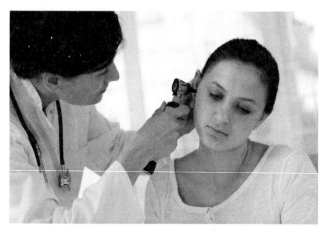

Step one of hearing test: external ear inspection.
Photo (c) gajdamak www.fotosearch.com

External or Outer Ear Evaluation

The first step of the hearing evaluation was a thorough check of my outer ears. The audiologist examined the outsides for redness and signs of injury or infection. Then she used a special instrument called an *otoscope* to inspect the ear canals and the tympanic membranes. She looked for any obvious malformations of the ear canals, obstructions, such as wax, signs of inflammation, infection, fluid build-up, bleeding, and perforation or scarring of the eardrums. It is not uncommon for children to have ear canals that are blocked by beads, peas, and all sorts of other edible or inert materials. In order for us to hear, however, and for hearing tests to be meaningful, sound must have a clear path for travel.

If the audiologist detects anything suspicious with the outer ear structures or eardrums, the patient's medical doctor is informed and decides on further evaluation and/or treatment. This might not be a good time for hearing tests. Both my outer ears and eardrums looked normal, and we got ready for the next step, the middle ear assessments.

Middle Ear Tests: acoustic immittance measures

Middle ear tests identify issues concerning the relay of sound vibrations. They begin with the visual inspection of the eardrums, and mine had already passed muster. For the subsequent evaluations, I did not have to do anything: the instrument recorded the findings, regardless of what I perceived or heard. A probe that felt like a snug plug was inserted into one ear and then the other. I was warned not to chew, talk, swallow, or move. Doing so would alter the ear canal air pressure and therefore interfere with the tests. The audiologist said I would feel pulses and hear brief buzzing sounds, but I did not need to respond.

Acoustic immittance measures are commonly administered for evaluating middle ear performance. In my case, they were done only once—during my initial hearing test visit. They included *tympanometry* and *acoustic reflex threshold* tests. Although they might not point to a definite cause for a hearing loss, these middle ear assessments provide important information for the physician.

Tympanometry evaluates the reaction of the eardrum and middle ear structures as they respond to rapid air pressure changes induced within the ear canal. The measurements are done with an instrument called a *tympanometer,* and the results for each ear are recorded on a graph called a *tympanogram.* A damaged, flabby, or stiffened eardrum; fluid accumulation or abnormal air pressure in the middle ear cavity; infection; a disconnect in the ossicle chain; middle-ear skin growths; a non-functioning eustachian tube; and otosclerosis, a stiffening of the stapes ossicle, all figure on the long list of reasons why tympanometry tests veer off base. I could feel my eardrums pulsate on both sides as a result of the pressure variations. It was a bit uncomfortable but not painful.

The *acoustic reflex test* detects stapedius muscle contraction in response to loud sounds. Does the muscle contract spontaneously as it should in a reflex-type manner? The softest sound that brings about such a reflex contraction is called the *acoustic reflex threshold* level. Again, the results for each ear are recorded on a separate grid. On the right side, I did hear the buzzing noises that were meant to elicit the desired muscle response, but I did not detect any sounds on the left side. I asked if this was a bad sign, but the audiologist did not seem alarmed and did not offer any comment. Later on, I found out that both my ears fell within normal limits for these tests. This was a rather traumatic time for me, and it would have been reassuring to have known that.

Inner Ear Tests: pure-tone audiometry

The next set of exams was designed to evaluate the response of my cochlear hearing cells to signals of different pitches or frequencies. This time I had to do the work while sitting in a soundproof booth. As the audiologist informed me, I was now the "key player." She handed me a clicker that I had to push whenever I heard a tone, no matter how faint. She stated that each ear would be tested separately and would get its own report.

As I sat down for these hearing checks, I was not only very tired but also rather upset and tense. I worried that I might not be able to concentrate well enough, which would affect the results. This was only my personal hunch, but I mentioned it to the audiologist. Unlike middle-ear measures, routine inner-ear hearing tests are not performed by unbiased, unemotional instruments. Instead, they are known to be *subjective* in nature, as it takes the full mental and physical cooperation of the patient for these assessments to be meaningful. The audiologist understood my trepidation. I was told that in order to neutralize that subjective bias, tests would be repeated. The future objective was to study a trend of my hearing performance.

The inner-ear evaluation process is commonly known as *pure-tone audiometry*. The term "audiometry" translates roughly as "hearing measurement." I have been told the expression "pure-tone" refers to the fact that the signals that are relayed to the patient during the tests consist of clean, crisp sounds, made of only one frequency at a time, unlike real-life noise that is more like a mixed-frequency salad.

The calibrated instrument used to administer the tests is called an audiometer; it registers the client's hearing sensitivity to sounds of different frequencies, or pitches. Pure-tone assessments are designed to determine how loud the individual signals must be for the ear to detect them. Hearing is evaluated over the frequency ranges that make up human speech. The pure-tone results are plotted on a graph called an audiogram.

There are two separate types of pure-tone tests: pure-tone **air** conduction and pure-tone **bone** conduction tests.

Pure-tone air conduction tests are usually done first. Here, computer-generated beeping sounds travel the standard way—through the air—from plug-type ear inserts or headphones through the ear canal to the eardrum through the middle ear to the cochlea. Cochlear hair cells then translate endolymph movements into electrical impulses that travel to the brainstem via the cochlear nerve.

In order to know what each ear *really* hears, the audiologist might mask the opposite ear with static noise. This keeps the non-test ear busy while its partner is being evaluated. *Masking* is particularly helpful if one ear is much weaker than the other one. During the assessment of the weaker ear, the test signals might have to be made loud enough for the healthier ear to actually perceive them. Masking reduces false-positive reports due to crossover of sound from one ear to the other. In essence, masking isolates the ear that is being tested.

For my pure-tone air conduction evaluation, the audiologist put small earplug-like probes into both my ears. Test beeps of different loudness and pitch were piped, first into one ear and then into the other. Whenever I heard a signal, I pressed the button on the clicker that I had been given. Patients can also be asked to notify the audiologist by giving a hand signal. As I reported my responses, the audiometer compared them automatically to those of a normally hearing population. The lowest volume that I detected for each test-frequency was determined to be my *threshold level,* or *hearing level,* for that particular frequency.

While my left ear was tested, my right ear was almost continuously masked. This is still done to this day, especially in the high-frequency area, where my hearing loss is most pronounced. The air-conduction tests administered during my first audiology visit showed that my right ear performed fine for my age. The left ear did not; I waited for signals. I knew that they were being sent. I strained to hear. I detected a couple of very low-pitched sounds. It was demoralizing to know that tones that were relayed to the ear did not register. After the pure-tone air conduction tests were finished, it was time for the pure-tone *bone* conduction series.

For **bone-conduction tests**, an oscillator presents the sound in *vibration* form. This time, the *skull bones* conduct the signals directly to the cochlea, where the vibrations cause endolymph movements. Again, the cochlear hair cells translate these motions into electrical impulses that travel to the brain by means of the cochlear nerve.

Bone conduction *bypasses* the outer and middle ears and isolates the cochlea. If the client's hearing scores are better with bone conduction than with air conduction, it can be assumed that the problem is associated with an outer and/or middle ear issue. Comparing the air-conduction and bone-conduction test results helps the specialist determine what type of hearing loss the patient might have and decide on further evaluations.

In preparation for these assessments, the audiologist removed the ear inserts from my ears. Then she strapped the oscillator, or vibrator, to the mastoid bone in back of my left ear. The oscillator was attached to a tight metal headband that held it in snug contact with the bone. She instructed me to listen for sounds and warned me that "feeling something, such as a tickle," did not count. The right ear was masked during the test. Unfortunately, my left ear did not detect any sound, and because it had already done very poorly with air conduction, further tests were halted. At this point, my ear could be described as being deaf, or at best, as having a profound hearing loss. Yet in spite of all the tests, I still had no idea *why* it was deaf—and that proved to be very unsettling.

ABR (auditory brainstem response) Test

As I went to my first audiology session, I had an inadequate general understanding of hearing tests. I certainly did not know the purpose or value of air and bone conduction assessments. Once it had been established that my left ear did not hear under any circumstance, I kept on worrying about nerve damage. I wondered if any of these evaluations had given an answer to that question. The following morning, I detected human voices on my hospital pillow speaker, a turn of events that was rated as "highly positive" by Dr. Todd. He mentioned that signals were getting through to the brain, which bode well for the cochlear nerve.

Later on, I learned about the *ABR* test (auditory brainstem response), which is also known as the *BAER* test (brainstem auditory evoked response). It evaluates the nerve pathways between the cochlea and the brainstem and is therefore helpful for verifying cochlear nerve function. It is one of the tests used for checking newborn babies' hearing and for assessing patients who are unable to cooperate with standard testing procedures. It can also be performed when working with clients whose hearing loss is believed to be related to nerve damage or problems due to stroke or tumors. The ABR is painless, and the patient does not have to respond to any signals.

Electrodes are placed on the earlobe, forehead, and scalp of the test side. Next, clicking sounds are delivered to the ear by means of a probe that is inserted into the ear canal. The electrodes detect brain activity evoked by these signals, and the audiologist's instruments record the brain's responses. In patients with cochlear nerve or brainstem damage, the brainstem's response to sound is abnormal or may be absent.

The OAE (otoacoustic emissions) Test

This non-invasive test evaluates cochlear hair-cell function. Together with the ABR, it is a standard test administered when checking newborn hearing or when evaluating patients who cannot be tested in conventional ways. No patient response is necessary.

The normal cochlea emits its own little noises, both at rest or when stimulated by sound. This cochlear "back talk" is known as "otoacoustic emissions." The sounds are believed to be produced by the outer cochlear hair cells, so named for their location within the cell lineup. Otoacoustic emissions are present in people with normal or close-to-normal hearing. They die down with aging and with hearing loss.

In order to perform the test, an ear insert equipped with both a loudspeaker and a microphone is placed into the ear canal. The loudspeaker relays a series of signals to the cochlea. In response to these sound stimuli, the cochlea sends forth very low-volume noises. These are picked up by the probe's microphone and analyzed by the audiologist's instruments. Cochlear emissions allow the audiologist to measure cochlear activity under different sound conditions.

Most Common Types of Hearing Loss

Defects that are related to the *outer* and/or *middle-ear* section(s) produce a **conductive hearing loss**. This means, the sound is not conducted properly and fails to travel efficiently through the air to the inner ear. The audiogram shows a sizeable gap between the air conduction and bone conduction test results. Bone conduction performance scores surpass the air conduction scores. Many problems that contribute to this type of loss can be treated or maybe repaired. Ultimately, hearing can be assisted with bone-conduction hearing aids, if traditional air-conduction devices are of little or no help.

A hearing decline related to the cochlea and the relay of signals to the brain results in **sensorineural hearing loss.** The term "sensori" refers to the cochlear hair cells. A number of these might be weak, damaged, or even dead at certain frequencies. Therefore, they respond poorly, or they do not respond at all, which leads to issues with sensing sound.

The word "neural" usually refers to the cochlear nerve but can also include other hearing or auditory nervous pathways. There are telltale signs that reveal to the audiologist whether the loss is more sensori or more neural in nature.

I have a sensorineural hearing loss—the most common type of hearing loss—in the high-end frequencies or pitches. Whichever of my cochlear cells are damaged or dead will remain so. So far, this kind of loss is permanent and irreversible. The best we can do is to make the most of the hearing that is left. Noise-induced hearing loss and to a large extent hearing loss of aging, or *presbycusis* are of this type.

People whose hearing loss involves both conductive and sensorineural issues have a **mixed hearing loss.**

Speech Audiometry

Normally, speech tests would have followed the bone-conduction series during my first audiology visit. As my left ear was deaf, none of these exams were performed on me until my follow-up appointment, three weeks after my ear event.

Speech audiometry tests provide a lot of valuable information for the specialists. They tell at what volume or loudness we *perceive* speech. They help establish loudness comfort and discomfort levels, which is important for calibrating hearing instruments. They also test *understanding* of speech, the biggest challenge of those with hearing loss, especially in background noise.

Three weeks after my initial tests I had a repeat hearing evaluation. This time, I felt that I did better. The audiologist stepped into the booth and informed me with controlled excitement that I had regained a modest amount of hearing. We would be able to add a *speech* evaluation test. My hearing, however, was still way too poor for me to try some of the more sensitive assessments—there would be none of the tests that involved different types of softly spoken material. No whispers for me. As it turned out, we never did any of those threshold tests, not then and not on subsequent visits. My hearing never improved to the point where my left ear could detect or understand low-intensity speech.

The *speech reception threshold (SRT)* test—one of the tests I was not given—is performed on each ear separately. Sitting in a soundproof booth, the patient listens to a voice speak two-syllable words. The challenge is to hear these words and to repeat them correctly as the voice decreases gradually in loudness. How low can the volume go for the patient to still identify the spoken words correctly at least 50 percent of the time? That faintest level is recorded as the speech reception threshold, or SRT.

The *speech detection threshold (SDT)* test—another test that I skipped—is also known as the *speech awareness threshold (SAT)*. This time the patient must detect speech. The exam determines the lowest sound volume for the patient to become aware of speech at least 50 percent of the time. This is a "Can you hear me now?" kind of a test which is totally out of my reach.

The test that the audiologist added during my follow-up hearing evaluation was the *word recognition* test, which used to be known as "speech discrimination" test. This assessment is now routinely included whenever I go for a hearing recheck. While sitting in the soundproof booth, I listen to one-syllable words, such as room, broom, air, pair, etc. Each word is spoken by a calm, recorded male voice at a loudness level that is comfortable for me. My ears are tested separately. My task is to repeat the spoken words correctly. The answers are either right or wrong; there is no partial credit.

Word recognition helps to separate what I hear from what I understand. The percentage of words that I answer correctly is my result or test score. For example, if I am given twenty words to repeat, and I come up with fifteen correct answers, my score would be 75 percent. On my first try, the left ear scored 28 percent. Considering that just three weeks before, the test was not even administered, as my left ear was deaf, such a colossal grade was certainly a cause for celebrating.

I am aware that my word recognition leaves a lot to be desired. I have even laughed at some of my answers. I knew they were wrong, but they struck me as sadly humorous. Frankly, some of the responses were guesses and still are. Yet I always feel good about myself if I get at least the *sense* of the words. This is just for my own self-confidence. If I say "room" instead of "rooms," I consider that a partial success, although I do not get a point for the answer.

As I have lost a lot of hearing in the upper frequencies, I have trouble detecting certain sounds, such as *s, th, f, k, t,* which lie in the higher-frequency ranges. Those of us with such sound voids might catch portions of words after which the "brain fills in" based on context. The results can be amusing—or not so amusing. I can usually guess that things are not quite right if the speaker's body language does not fit what I hear. I once had a hard time believing that a coworker would have sent "nasty mail" to people. As it turned out, he had sent a "mass email". Although we all misunderstand a word now and then, people with hearing loss misunderstand more frequently and consistently.

For many people, a lot rides on the word recognition reports, especially if accurate hearing is a requirement for their jobs. Letting the brain "fill in" words or meaning can lead to dangerous and sometimes embarrassing situations. I was not in a profession where I could afford to guess at sound-alike drug or patient names. I also cannot imagine an airline pilot, whose place of work is a stressful, noisy cockpit, with faulty word recognition—that could be tough.

Keeping a Sense of Humor

That said, word recognition jokes abound among the hard-of-hearing people, but only we can tell them. There is nothing funny about it, as I well know, but even under sometimes trying circumstances, it is important to keep a sense of humor.

Actress Gilda Radner's *Saturday Night Live* routine was based a bit on the misunderstanding of words. Who doesn't remember the beloved yet quirky *Roseanne Roseannadanna* (from *Saturday Night Live*) and her civic concerns? I recall a tirade that she delivered on "*violins*" on television. There was certainly nothing wrong with that, she argued. Why was everybody so upset about this particular topic? When she was informed that the issue had to do with "*violence*," not violins, she gave her classic reply: "Never mind!"

In the air-disaster satire movie *Airplane!,* the character of Dr. Rumack, played by actor Leslie Nielsen, must inform the captain that a large number of passengers have come down with food poisoning.

Says the captain, "*Surely*, you can't be serious." Answers Dr. Rumack, "I am serious, and don't call me *Shirley*!"

***

Before the Audiogram: Mind the Wax

Ear wax, or *cerumen*, is often cited as a cause for hearing loss. It is the easy answer to give to those who are worried about their hearing. In essence, ear wax plugs can lead to a conductive hearing loss, as sound no longer flows freely through the ear canal to the eardrum. The patient experiences a gradual hearing deterioration as the ear canal fills up ever so slowly. The ear begins to feel stuffy, and sounds seem distant and fuzzy. Upon sneezing, people with ear wax blockages often report hearing noises akin to the whistling of a tea kettle. Air can barely move through the clogged canal. Once the canal is totally impacted, the moment comes where most, if not all, hearing fades away. Sound simply cannot reach the eardrum anymore. Ringing or buzzing (tinnitus) in the ear might accompany the hearing loss.

I tend to wear earplugs in situations where I have little or no control over the noise levels. Earplugs, however, can push wax back down into the canal. My ENT doctor and audiologist had cautioned me not to overuse the plugs and to quit jamming them into the canal as far as possible; my technique was said to be overly aggressive. I heeded their words and thought that I had been careful, but in spite of my gentler approach I ended up with a "wax emergency."

One day I called Dr. Leonard's office in a panic. My right ear, my *good* ear, was causing me problems. It felt dull, and I experienced all sorts of swishing and whistling sounds. As usual, hearing tests had to be done before I saw the physician. The audiologist inspected the ears. She found a bit of wax on the left, but on the right there was a lot more. As an ear insert would have been lodged in the wax blockage, she used headphones for doing the hearing assessment. This time, I did show a hearing loss on the right ear.

67

Audiogram in hand, I showed up at Dr. Leonard's office practically in tears. I worried that this might be a replay of what had happened earlier on the left side. The doctor looked at the audiogram tracing and inspected the ear. This time, it was easy, he announced. I had a substantial wax obstruction in the right ear that he would remove. He inquired if had used cotton swabs for cleaning my ears—he thought that he saw some fibers. He informed me that in using such swabs, not only is the ear wax pushed backwards but more important, cotton fibers mix with the cerumen and turn it into a cement-like mass. The same is true for fibers from paper tissues. After the doctor cleaned both ears, my right-sided hearing returned to normal.

That day I was both relieved and upset—relieved that my good ear was fine after all, but upset that I had gone through yet another testing session, which is always traumatic for me. I ended up with an expensive audiogram—actually, more like a "wax-o-gram"—that was of no value and should not have been done. Although checking the integrity of the outer ear, which includes the ear canal, is the first step when doing a hearing assessment, I decided that I, the patient, would have to inquire about the ear wax situation whenever I had an audiogram done. If such a build-up threatened to bias the outcome, I would ask for it to be removed *before* any tests would be performed. That day, I also decided that I had to become a lot more knowledgeable in regard to hearing evaluations, so that I could act as my own watch dog. If I planned to be involved in my care, it was high time for me to learn.

Chapter 13
The Elements of an Audiogram

The results of pure-tone air and bone conduction tests, the backbones of hearing tests, are recorded on a chart called an audiogram. In these evaluations, hearing sensitivity of the person being tested is compared at different frequency or pitch levels to the sensitivity of a normally hearing population.

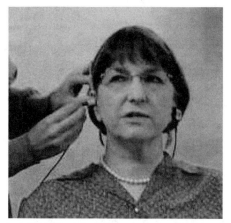

After the hearing test, the patient should receive an audiogram showing the results. If not-ask for it. *Photo R.Hammond*

The day after my ear event, my first audiogram showed that I was deaf in the left side. On subsequent visits, the reports became more informative for the specialists, but I had no clue what all the markings and squiggles were about. The whole matter was explained to me in one sentence: I had the typical downhill ski-slope pattern of a high-frequency sensorineural hearing loss. What did that mean? I did not expect anybody to give me a crash course in audiology, as I assumed that the explanations would be technical and lengthy. So, if I wanted to know more, I would have to find out for myself.

Pitch and Loudness

Two words dominate the conversation when people discuss their hearing tests: pitch and loudness. Although they refer to our *perception* of sound, these are not scientific terms. Yet specialists might use the expressions because they make sense to the patients. Pitch and loudness, however, reflect a personal or subjective bias that varies from person to person. What seems loud and painfully high-pitched to me might sound just fine to others. Our perception of a given noise is simply different.

Luckily, science has been successful in getting rid of the subjective slants that follow patients into the test cubicle. Audiology needs units of measurement that are defined, repeatable, and devoid of emotional baggage or personal prejudice. Therefore, expressions of pitch and loudness are not used. Instead, specialists talk about frequency and sound intensity or sound volume.

Frequency

In both physics and audiology, sound pitch is called "frequency." The unit used to measure frequency is the *hertz (Hz)*, named for the German physicist Heinrich Rudolf Hertz, who lived from 1857 to 1894. He was a physics professor with a particular love for the field of electromagnetism. He was also the first person to send and receive radio waves.

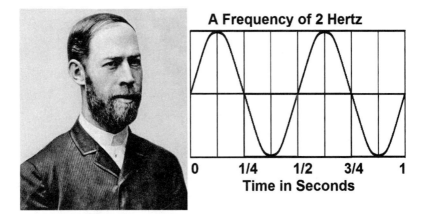

Heinrich Hertz and a Diagram of 2 Hertz, 2 cycles or two sound waves per second
*- photo:"Heinrich Rudolf Hertz" by Robert Krewaldt - Licensed under Public
Domain via Wikimedia Commons // Frequency diagram by Author*

Sound is made up of a continuous stream of waves that follow one another. The hertz tells us how many times per second a wave *cycles,* from its low point, or trough, to the peak and back down again. If only one wave is formed per second, the frequency would be 1 Hz; 5 waves per second 5 Hz; 100 waves per second 100 Hz, etc. The faster the waves follow one another, the faster their cycling pace per second, the higher their frequency. Waves that follow one another at a slower rate have a lower frequency; they have fewer cycles per second.

In real life, sound is made up of intermingling and superimposed sound waves of all sorts of frequencies. The useful thing about hearing tests is that our hearing is assessed in response to tones made of only *one* frequency. This allows the specialist to pinpoint where, within the testing range, there is a hearing issue. My loss starts in the mid-ranges but is worse for the high frequencies.

Approximate Frequency Ranges

As these are rather abstract notions, I found it helpful to check the frequencies for some familiar sounds. This gave me a sense of how hertz values translate into practice. For a properly tuned eighty-eight-key piano, the lowest key produces sound waves that cycle at about 28 Hz. This is a lingering, droning, very low sound. The highest piano note strikes up at about 4,100 Hz. The middle C key comes in at around 250 Hz. The voice range of a soprano lies between 250 and 1000 Hz. Normal human hearing can range from 20 to 20,000 Hz, but as we age, our hearing sharpness declines quickly, especially in the noisy world in which we live.

Pure-tone tests survey our hearing within the frequencies of *human speech*, starting at 250 Hz and going all the way to 8,000 Hz. Although the major speech frequencies are usually considered to top off around 4,000 hertz, I was told that higher-range hearing provides extra bonuses, such as richness, intelligibility, naturalness, and clarity. As high frequencies are lost, hearing becomes poorly defined and dull, and people complain that they have trouble understanding speech, especially in background noise. Suddenly, the difference between hearing and understanding becomes painfully obvious.

Sound Intensity, Sound Volume, and Hearing Level

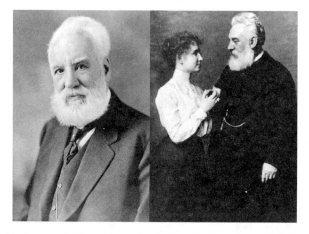

Alexander Graham Bell and Alexander Graham Bell together with Helen Keller
photos - Wikipedia / Moffett Studio / Library and Archives Canada / C-017335]
// "Helen Keller and Alexander Graham Bell" by Perkins School for the Blind
Archives - Own work. Licensed under CC BY-SA 3.0 via Wikimedia Commons /
*https://commons.wikimedia.org/wiki/File:Helen_Keller_and_Alexander_Graham_*
Bell.jpg#/media/File:Helen_Keller_and_Alexander_Graham_Bell.jpg // United
States Library of Congress's Prints and Photographs division Licensed under Public
Domain via Wikimedia Commons

When measuring sound loudness, things become a bit more complex. What we call "loudness" is better referred to as *sound intensity or sound volume,* which is measured in *decibels,* or *dB* (dee-bee). The dB is named for Alexander Graham Bell, the inventor of the telephone. More important for us, Mr. Bell was a teacher for deaf people. His own mother was very hard of hearing, and his wife, a former student, was deaf. He once tutored Helen Keller, who dedicated her autobiography to him.

The dB is a logarithmic unit of measurement; actually a ratio, where a given sound is compared to a reference sound. The dB tells us how many times louder or fainter a particular sound is than the given reference sound. Applying the notion of the decibel to human hearing tests turned out to be a challenge for scientists. The major obstacle to designing a standardized test format was in setting a reference sound intensity for each assessed frequency. Thanks to the ingenuity and efforts of audiologists and experts at the American National Standards Institute (ANSI), we have the *Hearing Level* scale, which offers a way to evaluate hearing in a reproducible, standardized fashion.

On the Hearing Level scale, the average softest hearing sensitivity of a normal-hearing population serves as the reference point for each frequency and is called the *normal threshold level*. For simplicity's sake, the value of the normal threshold level for each test frequency was arbitrarily set at 0 dB (zero decibels). Detecting sound at the 0 dB level indicates normal or good hearing.

During the tests, the patient's softest response for each test frequency is automatically compared by the audiometer to the average softest response of the normal population. The patient's score that is recorded on the audiogram as "Hearing Level" is the *patient's threshold level*. For example, if I am tested at the frequency of 1,000 Hz and I detect the beep at a volume of 45 dB, I am said to be 45 dB "down" at 1,000 Hz. In practice this means that the softest average intensity—0 dB—heard by a normal-hearing population at 1,000 Hz had to be increased to 45 dB for me to hear it. Therefore, my threshold level at 1,000 Hz is recorded as 45 dB on the audiogram hearing level scale.

Normal Hearing Range

If at each frequency the normal threshold level is 0 dB, what do the *negative* hearing level numbers on the audiogram mean? If one considers zero as normal, or good hearing, there will always be people who hear *better* than normal. This is expressed by a score in the negative values. "Normal" subjects, however, whose hearing is a tad less sensitive than the standard 0 db must also be accounted for. Although their hearing is very keen, their scores lie slightly below the 0 dB mark. Due to the great variation that exists among people, "normal human hearing" has been fitted into an acceptable *dB range*.

How tight that range should be is a matter of discussion and debate among specialists. It is usually felt that for every test frequency, the normal hearing sensitivity lies between -10 dB and +20 dB. This range was used for my audiograms. Upgraded, more stringent guidelines, however, reflect the position that normal hearing cannot be extended beyond 15 dB. The American Speech-Language-Hearing Association (ASHA) lists normal human hearing levels between -10 dB and +15dB.

Approximate dB Values

There are many sources that list the approximate sound intensity levels, expressed in dB, for various noises. In order to spare our ears from noise-induced hearing loss, it is a good idea to get an appreciation for how loud things really are.

Normal human conversation in a quiet environment measures about 60 dB, while a whisper is recorded at 30 dB. An average refrigerator hums along at 40 dB (though, honestly, mine must be a lot more). Moderate rainfall measures around 50 dB. A washing machine swishes and swashes at 75 dB.

Heavy city traffic pumps out some 85 dB, but it can also be a lot louder. A regular power lawnmower registers around 90 dB. I cannot imagine what those industrial, super-duper, dual- and triple-blade mower monsters put out, but I hope they come with an industrial-strength set of hearing protectors. An ambulance siren blares at 120 dB. Very loud, sudden, close-range noises, such as a jet engine at takeoff or a shot from a 12-gauge shotgun, have the potential for causing immediate, serious damage to the cochlear hair cells, maybe even deafness.

Lengthy exposure to 85 decibels and above warrants ear protection, as we are entering the hearing damage danger zone.

Examples of Pure-tone Audiograms

Two audiograms are shown below. The first graph details normal hearing, while the second graph shows the results of my third audiogram, done about three months after my sudden hearing loss incident.

Frequency listings in hertz (Hz) appear on the horizontal axis along the top. *Hearing level* values, expressed in dB, are on the vertical axis to the left. The starting point for every test frequency is the normal threshold of 0 dB. On these reproductions, all markings are in black. However, on original audiogram copies the tracings for the right ear are shown in red, while those for the left ear appear in blue.

As I mentioned earlier, nowadays our hearing is considered normal if we can hear test-tone frequencies ranging from 250 Hz to 8,000 Hz at a hearing level of 15 dB or less. At the time when my third test was done, 20 dB was considered to be within normal hearing limits, and many specialists still find this to be an acceptable "normal" value.

The legend explaining the test symbols is usually listed on the report sheet, along with the audiogram.

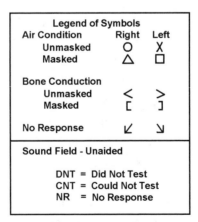

The Symbol Legend as it appeared on the author's Audiogram showing some of the standard symbols used when recording hearing tests. *diagram by Author*

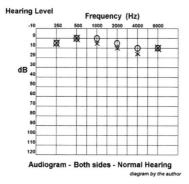

Audiogram - Both sides - Normal Hearing
diagram by the author

Audiogram No. 1 Hearing levels vary between ears, but audiogram
is within normal limits.

Audiogram # 1 shows unmasked, air-conducted right and left
ear responses. The hearing levels are all located within the acceptable
ranges of 20 dB or less. Both ears were tested between the frequencies
of 250 and 8000 hertz. This could easily represent my great hearing
before my ear event.

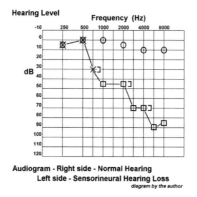

Audiogram - Right side - Normal Hearing
Left side - Sensorineural Hearing Loss
diagram by the author

Audiogram No.2 After the hearing loss the author had normal hearing
in the right ear but a steep hearing loss in the left ear.

As mentioned, audiogram No. 2 shows the results of the third
hearing test performed after my sudden hearing loss. The air-
conduction circles for my right ear all register within the range of -10

dB to 20 dB. The right ear was not tested with bone conduction, as it responded normally to air-conducted sound.

My left ear gave normal air-conduction responses at 250 Hz and at 500 Hz. The hearing loss becomes evident at around 750 Hz, where I am "down" by 30 dB. Starting at 1,000 hertz, the air-conduction results for my left ear were obtained while *masking* my right ear. I dip to 45 dB at 1,000 and 2,000 Hz; 70 dB at 3,000 and 4,000 Hz; 90 dB at 6,000 Hz; and 85 dB at 8,000 Hz.

As my right ear was masked, my left ear was tested with bone conduction at 750 Hz; 2,000 Hz; and 4,000 Hz. The bone-conducted responses for those frequencies almost coincided with the air-conducted scores. In other words, bypassing the outer and inner ear by means of bone conduction did not produce superior results. This finding, together with my tympanometry report, led to the conclusion that I did not have a conductive hearing loss. Instead, all indicators pointed to a sensorineural hearing loss—but nobody explained this to me at the time.

The plotted results for my left ear make the outline of a *downhill ski-slope* curve, typical for upper-frequency sensorineural hearing loss. A friend with *Ménière's* disease has the problem opposite to mine. He does not hear much in the low frequencies but improves in the higher ranges. He has the *uphill slope* configuration.

Hearing loss is often described in broad terms as affecting a certain frequency "range." People might be told that their audiogram shows a low-frequency loss, a midrange frequency loss, or a high-frequency loss. I have asked various audiologists how these ranges are defined. I learned that there are no clear guidelines for sectioning off the test frequencies. Although there is room for debate, in general, frequencies up to 750 Hz are considered to be in the low-frequency range, while those between 750 Hz to 1,500 Hz qualify as midrange. Frequencies above 1,500 Hz are the high frequencies. At least those are the most consistent responses that I obtained from specialists.

Chapter 14
Quantifying Hearing Loss

As patients, our ultimate question is how serious our hearing loss really is. There are various hearing-loss classifications in existence, and not all audiologists use the same ones. Some references consider values down to 20 and 25 dB as "normal hearing," while others include these levels in the "slight hearing loss" category. Tighter, less lenient groupings reflect the understanding that losses that may appear minor on paper can have a detrimental impact on our existence. For instance, even a mild hearing loss greatly affects children's ability to learn.

Numbers on audiograms are not sensitive to turmoil or pain. In reality, hearing is so much more than a collection of figures and classifications, which does not express how profoundly hearing loss can interfere with our quality of life in terms of undermining our self-confidence and creating emotional, social, professional, and financial hardships.

The commonly accepted ASHA (American-Speech-Language-Hearing Association) chart below gives an idea of how our hearing compares to the normal 0 dB reference point for each test frequency.

ASHA Chart showing Degree of Hearing Loss	
Normal hearing	-10 to 15 dB
Slight hearing loss	16 to 25 dB
Mild hearing loss	26 to 40 dB
Moderate hearing loss	41 to 55 dB
Moderate severe hearing loss	56 to 70 dB
Severe hearing loss	71 to 90 dB
Profound hearing loss	91dB +

ASHA Chart showing the Degree of Hearing Loss from the American
Speech-Language-Hearing Association

To explain a hearing loss, the most accurate way would be to cite the decibel loss at each frequency. This is a rather clumsy method, however, and means little to those who are not familiar with hearing tests in the first place.

I describe my loss over the frequency test range. Consulting my audiogram and the ASHA classification, I say that I have a left hearing loss that starts out as mild to moderate in the midranges and goes from moderate to severe in the high frequencies. For most people this explanation is still too lengthy and complicated. They want to boil down their test results to *one* clear number that summarizes how much hearing they have lost overall. Considering that hearing assessments are done over a whole range of frequencies, there really is not one neat expression that says it all. Yet many of us are creatures of few words who want to wrap our minds around this hearing loss bit—and audiology obliges.

The Audiology PTA Score

In order to come to a single value for describing hearing loss, audiologists calculate a pure-tone average (PTA) value for each ear. The obvious advantages are that the use of one score makes it easier for people to relate to their loss and to describe it to others. The PTA value expresses an *average dB loss,* not a *"percent" hearing loss.*

To determine the PTA value, the specialist adds the hearing level scores for three standard frequencies, divides that sum by three (because three frequencies were used), and comes up with an average dB loss, or PTA, for the specified ear. For the PTA calculation, the frequencies of 500, 1,000 and 2,000 hertz are routinely used because they are considered to be major speech frequencies. The frequency of 3,000 hertz, however, can also be added; it all depends.

As patients, we should know how our PTAs are calculated, which frequencies are chosen to do so, what the numbers express, and into which hearing-loss category each ear fits. For example, if a patient's hearing level for the right ear is 40 dB at 500 Hz, 50 dB at 1,000 Hz, and 60 dB at 2,000 Hz, the decibels are added together (40 + 50 + 60) for a total of 150 dB. In order to arrive at the PTA value, the decibel sum is divided by 3 (150 ÷ 3) for an average of 50. In this case, the PTA score for the right ear is 50 dB, which expresses an average 50 decibel hearing loss over the three chosen frequencies. According to the ASHA chart, the patient has a moderate hearing loss in the right ear.

In a way, the standard PTA frequencies discount the contribution that higher-end frequencies make to relevant and intelligible speech. There is, however, so much more to hearing and understanding in complicated noise environments than "detecting sound" on three frequencies in a soundproof booth.

Other Uses for the PTA

Besides providing the patient with an average decibel hearing-loss score, the PTA helps audiologists with diagnostic decisions. Insurance companies, government agencies, and human resource departments also use PTA values when calculating a "hearing handicap" in compensation cases or employment-related situations. These financial, risk, and efficiency specialists use patient audiogram results, along with complicated formulas, to estimate the *percent* impairment, or disability, caused by a person's hearing loss. Based on their findings, they conclude how fully productive a client still is or what *percentage* disability insurance or pension he/she can claim. In work-related situations, hearing handicap assessments might help determine whether an employee continues to work in the current capacity; whether he/she should be reassigned to a different duty; or whether he/she qualifies for disability benefits.

The *degree of hearing loss* expressed in dB by the PTA score and the *percentage of disability* that results from a loss are two different issues that must be kept separate. It is important for us to understand these differences, if we are to argue our case with human resource representatives or insurance agents in a knowledgeable way.

***

Bridging the Communication Gap

Ideally, patients should check on their hearing test results with the doctor or audiologist before leaving the office. Although there are all kinds of issues to be discussed, it is amazing how many people know frightfully few details regarding their evaluations. In order to learn more about their hearing loss and the significance of their test scores, however, patients must communicate actively with their hearing specialists. Unfortunately, clients often do not ask enough (or any) questions, and the experts might not offer more than the bare minimum of information. The end result is an acute failure to communicate that disengages patients from their care.

Whenever we visit our regular doctor, most of us want to look at our blood test results, at our scan or x-ray pictures. In audiology, for some reason, we are more willing to be satisfied with few details. Maybe we are just spooked by an alien world we have been forced to enter without advance education. So far, there is no *Ear ER* TV show to introduce us to the concepts of hearing and hearing loss and to turn them into household words.

From our point of view as patients, many obstacles can get in the way of our asking questions. We might be scared of the truths that our tests reveal. We might be emotionally upset and in no condition to open up a dialogue with the ear specialist. All of this certainly applied to me at the time of my first audiology session. I was overwhelmed, and the minimum amount of information was all that I could handle. I simply did not want to see the bad news all plotted out for me on a piece of paper.

One of the greatest challenges in health education is to evaluate how much the patient can absorb, especially on a first visit. Most people, however, gradually emerge from their initial state of shock, fear, anger or, seeming disinterest. They are ready to talk.

I was prepared to ask some questions when I went back for my second set of hearing tests and follow-up visit with the doctor. I had become worried that the extreme noise exposure at the church might have jostled my middle ear ossicles or caused damage to the miniscule muscles. I was fixated on the idea that middle ear damage had made me deaf. Although I was appeased that this was not true, I was offered few insightful details.

During yet another follow-up evaluation, however, an audiologist told me that my left middle ear had tested normal. She mentioned sort of as an aside that "both my middle ears looked good." When I wondered how she could tell, she said, "From the test results, of course." She pointed out that the tympanometry and acoustic reflex reports were within normal limits. Also, my bone conduction scores did not suggest middle ear damage. Aha, those wavy lines, markings, and numbers actually did provide information to the trained eye on middle ear function.

The turning point that convinced me to get involved in my care came with the wax-o-gram episode, when my right ear—my good ear—was assessed when it was full of wax. Naturally, the ear registered a loss, as the wax was not cleared from the ear canal before the test was done. This experience both scared and frustrated me. I was, however, mostly upset at myself for my lack of engagement. That day, I decided to learn on my own, to question any specialist involved with my care, to insist on answers that I could understand, and to take the lead in my personal ear and hearing education program. Amazingly enough, my new approach made professionals more talkative. My showing knowledge of some basic audiology elements opened the door to more informative discussions.

It is indeed important for us to get explanations regarding our hearing status, especially since we often must be our own best advocates. If we remain uninformed, others will make life-altering decisions for us, without any input of our own.

There are many advantages to bridging the communication gap with our specialists. By getting a clearer understanding of our condition, we will be better able to cope and adjust, which in turn empowers us in many ways. Whenever we are ready to learn, it is time to say: "Show me the tests, and let me have the facts." And we must insist upon it.

Chapter 15
The Many Causes of Hearing Loss

As I sat in the chair at the ear, nose, and throat (ENT) clinic on the morning after my hearing loss, Drs. Leonard and Todd peppered me with plenty of open-ended questions. Their goal was to get a thorough ear and overall health history. They looked for any hints that could lead them toward a diagnosis or a plausible explanation for my predicament. The list of possible causes for hearing loss is a long and complicated one. The most frequently cited reasons, however, emerged from the inquiry to which I had to submit on that dismal day.

Ear canal problems

Both the emergency room physician and the audiologist had certified that my ear canals were obstruction-free. The flow of sound to the eardrums was not hampered by wax impactions, canal malformations, or signs of infection.

Excessive noise

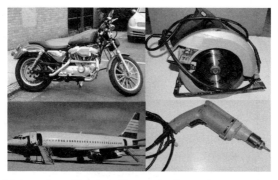

Motorcycles without mufflers, noise from a jet, power saws and drills can all exceed 100 dB. *photos: R.Hammond*

Drs. Leonard and Todd were most intrigued that a loud noise exposure preceded my hearing loss event. They felt that it more than likely aggravated the damage from an underlying viral infection and therefore greatly contributed to my issues. Exposures to excessively loud sound eventually poison the hair cells in the cochlea and erode their connections to the hearing nerve. The louder the noise, the shorter the exposure time before harm occurs, especially if there is already a predisposition. That day, I might very well have received a double dose of trouble. Some people think that loud noise is cool and fun. The amplifier maniacs at that church fundraiser most likely felt that way, never giving a thought to the fact that they might actually damage people's ears.

In my family I knew of two cases of noise-induced hearing loss. My father acquired a hefty loss due to his own negligence. He did not believe in using ear protection when doing target-practice shooting. My grandfather, a schoolteacher, also used to cup his ear in order to hear more efficiently. The daily grind of tending to noisy kids in a one-room school probably had something to do with his hearing problems. Years of church choir practice punctuated by energetic organ crescendos did not help him either.

Eventually, the doctor told him that he had a condition known as *presbycusis*, which translates loosely as "elderly hearing." As we age, our often already damaged cochlear cells become less sensitive and hearing declines as a consequence. Presbycusis is a progressive sensorineural hearing loss that affects both ears. It is brought on by the aging process and a lifetime of wear and tear, a good portion of which is noise-related. Also, cardiovascular issues, which may lead to a decrease in blood flow to the brain and ears, can further contribute to the problem. As the brain adapts to the gradual loss, people might not even notice that their hearing is fading out … until, one day, they feel that everybody mumbles and that they are excluded from conversations.

Vascular issues

On the morning of my first ENT visit, Dr. Todd and I discussed the possibility of an "ear stroke." Good blood irrigation is needed to maintain adequate oxygen levels, which are essential for peak cochlear performance. Yet the cochlea is not equipped with an extensive network of blood vessels. Any interruption in blood flow to the ear, no matter how brief, can result in hearing loss. Dr. Todd wondered if a stress-induced blood vessel spasm might have been an added contributing factor in my case. Yes, I did have stress that day, which certainly could have worked against that already compromised left ear. He also mentioned that people who suffer a stroke of the brain may experience hearing loss, depending on the extent and location of the insult.

Although tests did not reveal any answers, I considered the mere possibility of a vascular event as a warning shot across the bow. In the interest of preserving the hearing I had left for as long as possible, I became seriously motivated to clean up my diet and lifestyle. With my doctor's consent, I put myself on a regular exercise schedule. I attempt to manage stress, which is a real challenge for me, and eat plenty of fruits and veggies. By now, the sheer mention of trans fats makes me cringe. There might not be any guarantees, but I do my best not to sacrifice my hearing to artery-choking plaque.

Family history

Leading with the comment that we "are our genes," Dr. Leonard then launched into a series of questions on my family health and hearing histories. Hearing disorders can indeed be *genetic* in nature, but I did not know of anyone in my family who had been born deaf or hard-of-hearing or who had ear malformations of any kind.

The doctors wondered if any of my blood relatives experienced off-and-on episodes of dizziness and hearing loss. They were thinking of *Ménière's disease.* I knew of the condition but was not intimately familiar with the details. Dr. Todd gave me the highlights: At first, it usually affects one ear. It seems to be linked to ear-fluid pressure problems. It often comes on without warning in attacks not unlike mine. In some cases, evidence shows a family connection. I was relieved to say that I had no knowledge of such issues among my kin. Of course, that did not mean that I could not be affected. The doctors concluded that we would wait and see if further episodes would follow. Time would tell.

The question whether any of my blood relatives had ever needed ear surgery took me by surprise. Although I could not think of anyone, I wondered about the meaning of the question. Dr. Todd explained that the mention of "ear surgery" hints at family ear problems that must be clarified. For example, in severe cases of Ménière's disease special surgical procedures could have been performed in order to bring relief. Certainly, anatomic malformations might have been corrected or alleviated by surgical intervention.

The doctors, however, were considering the possibility of *otosclerosis*. This condition affects the middle ear and has a genetic connection in roughly 60 percent of the cases. The stapes, or stirrup ossicle, becomes fixed and can no longer relay vibrations to the inner ear. Otosclerosis leads to a slowly progressing hearing loss. Initially, patients can be helped with hearing aids, but as the stapes becomes less and less mobile, hearing worsens. During a surgical procedure known as a *stapedectomy*, the ossicle is removed and replaced with a prosthesis. Among my relatives, there had never been any cases of otosclerosis.

Next the doctors wanted to know if any of my family members suffered from rheumatoid arthritis (RA), systemic lupus erythematosus (SLE), multiple sclerosis (MS), or other conditions that I recognized as autoimmune disorders. I could not think of anybody who had complaints of that nature, although I wondered how autoimmunity could affect the ear.

With autoimmune disorders, the body essentially attacks itself. The natural defense system recognizes parts of the body as "foreign," assaults them, and begins to destroy them. Underlying genetic components are suspected, as autoimmune conditions tend to run in families. What ultimately unleashes the outbreak of a condition, or why the body gets trapped into making such self-abusive misjudgments in the first place, is still mostly unclear.

Although rare, direct immune attacks on the ears themselves are certainly known to happen. They result in *autoimmune inner ear disease* (AIED), which normally affects both ears. Symptoms can develop fast over weeks or months, or slowly over a year or longer. They include a progressive, often fluctuating hearing loss that can be accompanied by tinnitus, dizziness, and balance problems. If both ears are involved, hearing loss is often reported as being asymmetric, which means it is more severe in one ear than in the other.

In autoimmune reactions, besieged tissues or organs might not have been the primary targets of an attack. Instead, they may have become affected as a result of immune battles fought elsewhere in the body. In this case, immune by-products are carried by the bloodstream to different areas of the body, such as the ears, where they trigger trouble. Regardless of whether the ears are the intended targets or simply innocent bystanders, damage from any kind of immune assault is always serious, as it has the potential to destroy our hearing. So far, there are no specific tests to identify autoimmune ear disease, but doctors can get some helpful insights from hearing assessments, patient history, MRI scans, and from blood tests.

It reassured me that, as far as I knew, there were no autoimmune conditions in my family, yet the doctors did not take any chances. They added a whole litany of blood tests to an already impressive list. The MRI had yet to be done. This was so unsettling. Eventually, we got off the autoimmune topic and moved on to discuss other possible reasons for my woes. Incidentally, once all the test results were reported, it was decided that my ear had not come under attack by a misguided, confused immune system.

Ototoxic medications or substances

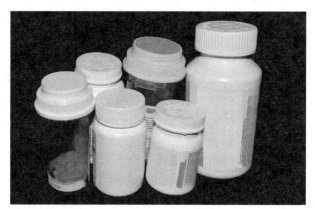

Certain medications and chemicals can be ototoxic. *photo: R.Hammond*

The doctor tag team now wondered if I had been sick recently or if any new medications had been prescribed for me. When the answer to both questions was no, I then had to recite all the medications, vitamins, supplements, or other health products that I was taking at the time. Luckily, it was a short list. They asked if I worked with any new chemicals at my job, or if I had been exposed to environmental toxins. They even inquired about insect bites. I was aware of the problems regarding ear-noxious substances, but I did not feel that my troubles were linked to them in any way. In the end, the doctors agreed with me.

The topic of ototoxicity is tremendously convoluted and stirs up a lot of controversy among professionals and patients alike. Chapter 17 discusses these issues further.

Head trauma

I was asked if I had sustained any recent head injuries, but I could not remember a blow or a fall of any kind. Head injuries can indeed cause havoc to the ear: perforation or tears in the eardrum, breaks in the boney cavity that protects the ear, disruption of the ossicle chain, and damage to the hearing and balance organs. Luckily, my follow-up MRI did not show any structural damage.

The question about head trauma, another preventable cause of hearing loss, made me wonder about all of those "healthy" contact sports. Now, when I see football tackles or kids being knocked onto the ice or into the guard wall during hockey games, or when I see wrestlers pin each other to the ground contorted like pretzels, I wonder. I wonder not only about their brains, bones, and spines but especially about their ears and their hearing. "Oh, they wear helmets," we say.

Infections

The doctors already had determined that I did not have an external ear infection. I had no signs of a bacterial middle-ear infection either. The eardrum looked pristine. Overall, they suspected that a viral invader might have played a part in my current condition. I was not amazed that today, in the "age of the virus," doctors routinely check people with sudden hearing loss for viral culprits, including HIV. Many infectious agents that we do not associate directly with the ears, however, can cause hearing loss. Viral diseases like mumps, measles, and German measles, and viral or bacterial meningitis are only a few examples. Middle-ear scarring due to chronic bacterial infections may lead to a conductive hearing loss.

Hearing loss related to neglected ear infections is often detected in older people who grew up when there were few antibiotics and when trips to the doctor were an exception rather than a rule. An audiologist once told me that she had seen eardrums in older patients that were so stiffened and scarred from lingering and repeat infections that she was not surprised by the outcome; namely, hearing loss that sometimes bordered on deafness.

Although doctors now tend to be more cautious about prescribing antibiotics, symptoms pointing to an ear infection are always a matter of concern. Before using the excuse that "nothing will be done anyway," it is best to have the situation checked out. The physician is the one who decides whether or not any infection must be treated.

Syphilis

In the course of my conversation with the doctors, it was mentioned that blood tests, including a screening for syphilis, were still pending. Although syphilis, the well-known scourge, has made a comeback, I had to think why such a test was needed, but then it all made sense. The long-term effect of syphilis of the ear, or *otosyphilis,* can produce a variety of inner ear symptoms. Dr. Leonard mentioned that in cases like mine, a syphilis screen was standard procedure. Vertigo, an intense spinning sensation, accompanied by a sudden severe hearing decline or even deafness could well be symptoms of a smoldering, late-stage syphilis infection.

One of the worrisome issues is that in the beginning stages, when it is easily treatable, symptoms are often vague or even absent. It is entirely possible that someone might not know that he or she contracted the disease at some point in life.

Patients can get very upset when they find out that they were tested without their knowledge for syphilis. Doctors, however, are simply searching for answers to our problems. So, it is nothing personal; it's just science.

Growths and tumors

According to Dr. Todd, the MRI of the head would look for tumors—any kind of tumors. He had already given the all-clear to abnormal skin growths, or cysts, of the middle ear, known as *cholesteatoma.* Cholesteatoma can be congenital in nature, which means that people are born with them. They may also develop as a consequence of a chronically malfunctioning eustachian tube and eardrum perforations due to chronic infections or direct trauma. Symptoms normally include off-and-on bouts of ear drainage, chronic ear drainage, feelings of fullness, and eventual hearing loss.

Cholesteatoma do not have any blood supply. Once they become infected, antibiotic treatment often brings little relief because the drugs are unable to penetrate the growths. They are surgically removed in order to prevent them from expanding and causing erosion of the ossicles and other destruction of the middle ear and beyond. This is one more reason why patients with infected, oozing ears are best evaluated by a specialist who can make sense of symptoms that might be easily mistaken for some other condition.

Dr. Todd referred to the potential tumors that interested him in my case as s*chwannomas.* He did not elaborate, but my curiosity was piqued, and I would find out more about these benign, silent nerve invaders shortly (see chapter 19). The doctors then reminded me of my upcoming MRI. After they left, I sat in the chair, and gradually it dawned on me that a brand new life was about to start: my life as a hard-of-hearing person.

Chapter 16
Noise-Induced Hearing Loss (NIHL)

Hearing loss has many causes over which we have little or no control. We cannot change our genetics. We cannot avoid every lurking virus or bacteria. We cannot command our immune system to behave. However, we often do have control over noise, the archenemy of our cochleae and hearing nerves. Noise-induced hearing loss (NIHL) is *preventable,* but it is also *permanent* and *cumulative.* From birth to death, no excessive noise insults are forgotten or forgiven.

Although sudden, explosion-type noise can cause immediate damage, NIHL is the result of repeated, prolonged exposures to overly loud sound. As the cochlear hearing cells and their connections to the hearing nerve suffer from decibel barrages, the signals that travel from the cochlea to the brain become progressively weak and unclear and therefore hard to sort out. One day, we feel that others mumble. We have trouble understanding speech in background noise. We misunderstand and misinterpret what is said. As the damage to the hearing structures and nerve pathways progresses, it also becomes increasingly difficult to get satisfactory results from hearing aids. Once noise-induced hearing loss has taken hold, it is tremendously important to learn about prevention strategies so that further damage can be avoided.

The healthy ear has a built-in system to protect itself from occasional, potentially harmful sounds. However, unrelenting, abusive noise assaults easily overpower Mother Nature's defenses. Every system has its limits.

The general attitude has been to tag hearing loss as an "old folks" condition, but rising noise levels have broken down age barriers worldwide. The World Health Organization (WHO) issued a statement warning of the threat to people's hearing due to excessive recreational and social sound levels. Over a billion teenagers and young adults are at risk across the world.

For children, the foundation for NIHL is often laid by noisy toys in overly noisy homes. Hearing specialists talk more and more about "young people with old ears." Also, the many veterans who come home from war duty, plagued by hearing damage and tinnitus, can be added to the NIHL list.

The Treacherous Onset of NIHL

As already stated, very loud, sudden noises can lead to immediate serious ear damage or even deafness. It came as both a shock and a surprise when I learned that lingering for too long in an obnoxiously loud environment played its part in my hearing loss. Generally speaking, however, noise-induced hearing loss is a treacherous, sneaky injury that happens slowly, over time. Tinnitus (ear noise) is often the first alarm signal that all is not well with one's hearing. Unfortunately, it takes a while to detect that a decibel here and there has been lost. As sounds gradually weaken and become distorted, music seems dull, and people start having serious communication difficulties. Then, they may be told that their audiogram shows irreversible high frequency losses, which cause their hearing challenges. Therefore, the time to become hearing-wise on noise is right now. Prevention is key.

Noise, Noise Everywhere

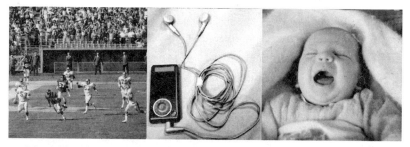

Many things in life can be too loud for unprotected ears. Stadium noise, MP3 players or even baby screams up-close, all can exceed 100dB. *photo: R.Hammond*

As a people, we contribute generously to the ear-noxious din that surrounds us. Our noise-hungry society is fascinated by the destructive forces of excess decibels. Movies are played back at insanely loud sound levels. Why might they crank the volume up so high? I was told that "the sound is part of the cinema experience." One does not only watch a movie, one also needs to "feel" it. If I understand this correctly, we are willing to kill off our ears for a few fleeting adrenaline rushes.

Why do some motorcycle enthusiasts remove the muffler from their machines? For some, it is simply "fun" to rev the engines and blast unsuspecting passersby with ear-numbing roars from the tailpipe. Unfortunately, they mostly blast themselves in the process.

More and more restaurants are excessively noisy. Kitchens and bars are incorporated into the dining areas, and noise-absorbing building materials seem to be things of the past. Piped-in music, mingled with the rattling of pots and pans and the clanking of dishes, blares away to the point where diners must yell at each other to be heard. Way too loud! Wait staff crouch down next to the tables in order to be at lip level with the customers. As a patron, I can leave. Employees, of course, must stay. Some restaurant reviewers now include dining room noise ratings as part of their reports on their

97

culinary experiences.

We can also encounter dangerous sound levels in places where we least expect them—like at church fundraisers, as I found out. Gyms are coming increasingly under attack for serving up aerobics and *Zumba* classes with hefty doses of ear-harmful decibels. Noise is everywhere, and we must become aware of that.

Rather than being fun, entertaining, and even youthful, loud noise turns out to be poison to the ears. It ages ears prematurely, which sets us up for a chronic communication disorder, called hearing loss. Hopefully, at some point, we will gain enough insight and maturity to understand that it is time to *turn down the volume.*

Perception is Not Reality

There is a sizable difference between our *perception* of a noise level and an *actual* instrument measurement. Physics and human hearing do not match up. People who work in acoustics are well aware that the brain can be an unreliable noise estimator. A *tenfold* increase in sound volume—as measured by an unbiased instrument—is perceived by the brain as being only about *twice* as loud as the previous level. The gap between actual sound intensity and our perception of it is mostly caused by a phenomenon known as *auditory adaptation.* Other psychological features, such as our emotions and our like-and-dislike bias, also play a part in how we perceive and evaluate sound volume.

Auditory adaptation is the brain's way of making everyday noises tolerable to us. Without it, we would probably be unable to adjust to such things as new sounds, changing sounds, or to the continuous variations in overall sound levels. Under normal circumstances or for as long as we operate in the no-danger decibel zones, this is certainly a good feature.

However, once we experience excessive noise levels, adaptation can easily lull us into a false sense of security by letting us believe that our sound environment is quieter than it actually is. The danger is that we become convinced to linger longer or to crank the stereo up another notch or two, any of which take the ear assault to the next level. Scientists tell us that this feeling of "desensitization" is a sign of Nature trying to protect itself from harm. Therefore, unsafe sound levels seriously endanger cochlear hair cells and hearing nerves, no matter what we "perceive." The end result is permanent hearing loss.

Those who function regularly in clamorous surroundings often report that they have gotten "used to" previously bothersome noise levels when in reality they have already lost hearing. In order to compensate for the hearing decline, overall higher sound volume levels are now needed. Gradually, people lose all sense of how loud things really are. One hearing downshift is followed by another, until a measurable noise-induced hearing loss becomes an obvious reality. In short: ears do not get "used" to loud sound or become "immune" to loud sound—at any age. They only become deafer to it.

Certainly, our personal bias of "like and dislike" also slips into the equation when we decide how loud might be *too loud*. It is easy to walk away from blaring music that is uninspiring to us, but *if we like* the music—even though we know that it is way too intense—we are tempted to stay and listen. We tell ourselves that the volume is not that bad and gradually, the infamous desensitization plays into our hands to the detriment of our ears. This is the problem with loud concerts and other entertainment. We attend specifically because we *like* the tunes, and this makes us careless. While we are busy deluding ourselves, cochlear cells are plowed under by the din, and their nerve connections become frayed. By the end of the "fun," the ears feel numb, hearing is dull, and we might experience tinnitus, or ringing in the ears—all symptoms pointing toward potential hearing damage that will hopefully become our wake-up alarm.

***

Avoiding Noise-induced Hearing Loss
Five Easy Actions

Various factors contribute to NIHL: the actual ear-level sound intensity, our proximity to the noise source, and the length of exposure. Basically, there are five easy things that we can do in order to protect our hearing from decibel assaults:

- We can *turn down the volume* or ask for the volume to be turned down.

- If that is not an option, we can put some *distance* between ourselves and the noise source by seeking out a quieter corner away from the loudspeakers.

- We can *leave* the situation altogether, which is probably the smarter choice.

- We can *limit* our exposure time—the shorter the better. The danger is that the longer we contemplate our options, the more our brain adapts and the more we lean toward suppressing our gut feeling that told us to get out of there in the first place.

- Especially, when we have little control over the sound environment, the most important step we can take is to use appropriate ear *protection*—earplugs or headphones, preferably the noise-reducing kind, in a timely fashion. On that notorious day, I eventually found some earplugs and used them but under the circumstances, I had waited too long. Yet, I learned my lesson.

Nowadays, I carry earplugs for all occasions at all times; I do not leave the house without them. My noise-reducing headphones have become my trusted travel companions. If only I had been blessed with such wisdom years ago!

Sound Levels and Exposure Times

When it comes to sound intensity, ignorance is not bliss. As we know, the brain can easily lead us astray in noisy situations. For our own safety, we must have at least some appreciation for *true*

100

decibel values as we head into a loud environment or work with loud equipment or tools.

In order to get an estimate of how loud a place might be, we can consult charts published by organizations, such as the National Institute for Occupational Safety and Health (NIOSH), or we might take a reading with our *smartphone app*. Noise levels at or above 85 dB move us into the danger zone for hearing damage. This means that we must take action and protect our ears. Power tools list prominently within the decibel range that calls for ear protection.

My personal rule is that if something seems too loud at first, it is. I still blame myself for not following my initial instinct—to make a quick exit—when the offensive cacophony overwhelmed me in that church hall. Of course, other forces might have been at work on my inner ear, and maybe it would not have made a difference if I had removed myself from the noise, but I will never know and I must accept that. If the noise makes us cringe, if we must yell in order to be heard by those standing next to us, *it is way too loud*.

Besides sound intensity, exposure time limits are a major concern. In the end, the question is: how loud is it and how long can we linger in the din? Again, we can consult the exposure time charts put out by the National Institute for Occupational Safety and Health (NIOSH), a part of the Centers for Disease Control and Prevention (CDC), or by the Occupational Safety and Health Administration (OSHA). OSHA is a US federal regulatory agency. For industry and the workplace, OSHA regulations are the law and command compliance. NIOSH is *not* a regulatory agency; it issues recommendations for best practice.

Noise exposure time limits and guidelines are *not guaranteed absolutes* that alone will protect us from noise-induced hearing loss. Numbers do not replace common sense and personal responsibility. Checking sound level and exposure time listings, however, raises awareness that too much noise for too long puts unprotected ears in harm's way pretty quickly. Once we reach the *maximum daily noise dose,* we must listen for the rest of the twenty-four hours to sound levels that are not in the harmful range—below 85dB. The ears simply need a rest. If they are not given that rest, we will pay the bill in currency of quality of life sooner rather than later.

Noise Exposure Time Limit for 24 Hours	Examples - for un-protected ears	
Noise or Sound	Level in dB	Time Limit
Quietest Sound for Normal Hearing	0	no limit
Normal Talking	60	no limit
Lunchroom / Cafeteria	85	8 Hours
SAFE NOISE LIMIT	85	8 Hours
Truck Traffic	90	2 Hours
Motorcycle	100	15 Minutes
Power Saw	110	90 Seconds
Siren / Concert	120	9 Seconds
Gun Firecracker *(immediate damage possible)*	*140+dB*	0 Seconds

Sources: NIOSH (National Institute for Occupational Safety and Health) and dangerousdecibels.org

Also, NIOSH has a fun, sound-enabled webpage for checking on noise levels and exposure times, called the *Noise Meter*. It particularly targets power tools and equipment. Give it a try at http://www.cdc.gov/niosh/topics/noise/noisemeter.html

OSHA has upgraded its mandated noise safety guidelines for the workplace. It now takes a more conservative approach than it did with earlier regulations. If unprotected ears are exposed to average daily noise levels of 85 dB for an eight-hour period, OSHA mandates that employers establish a "Hearing Conservation Program." This includes, among other requirements, the provision of appropriate ear protection free of charge, noise reduction efforts, such as equipment sound insulation, and the institution of sound level monitoring. Employees also must participate in yearly training programs on the effects of noise on ears and in the proper use and care of protective gear. Employers must make sure that hearing conservation guidelines are observed and enforced.

If 85 dB and above delineate the risk zone at the workplace, the same limits apply to our daily social and leisure activities. Nature does not care where the noise comes from. In the end, sound level and exposure time data may guide us, but only our protective actions and common sense will keep us safe.

Hearing Protection

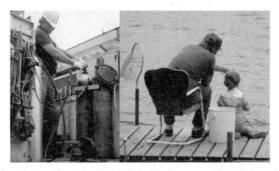

Industrial employees who work in loud areas need ear protection. Why risk not hearing one's grand-children? *photos: R.Hammond*

Avoiding excessive noise exposures altogether or reducing their impact by physical means are probably our best, immediate defenses against noise-induced hearing damage. Earplugs are an easy, affordable and portable solution for shaving some decibels off the din, but they are not appropriate for all. Earplugs tend to make the ear canal moist and itchy. They can also push wax back into the canal, especially if they are applied regularly or with too much vigor, as I learned. Patients with ear pressure issues, those who already have hearing loss, those who are prone to ear infections, or those who have problems with earwax or canal distortion do best to *consult with an audiologist* for the wisest ear-protection options in loud situations. In some cases, noise-dampening earmuffs might be a more acceptable alternative.

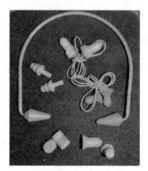

There are many of types of ear plugs, but ear plugs must be applied
correctly for maximum protection. *photo: R.Hammond*

It is amazing how many different styles and types of plugs are
available—sports plugs, air travel plugs, industrial plugs, musicians'
plugs, snore-blocking plugs, all-purpose plugs, etc. Earplugs
serve different purposes, depending on their shape, noise-filtering
characteristics and on the materials that they are made of. The latter
is important information for people with allergy issues. As there are
almost unlimited choices for any circumstance, it is worth taking
a look at the different types and styles of plugs available in stores,
catalogs or online.

For maximum protection, earplugs and earmuffs must be
correctly fitted and applied and consistently worn in loud places. They
carry a noise reduction rating (NRR) that tells by how many decibels
they can cut sound levels. My all-purpose plugs have an NRR value
of 32 dB—as long as I use and insert them *according to manufacturer
directions*. Unfortunately, most people never check on the instructions
for inserting earplugs properly and therefore will never come close to
the listed NRR values.

For professional musicians, who are exposed for hours and
hours to loud environments, audiologists can make custom-designed
earplugs. Of course, these are a lot more sophisticated than the
standard editions and can be somewhat pricey. Yet they do not clip

frequencies or distort sound. For dedicated concert-goers, it might be worthwhile to check on these new ways to protect ears while retaining sound quality.

Noise-cancelling headphones are a more expensive and visible choice. Sounds are neutralized or reduced by the production of sound waves of equal but opposite quality. My husband gave me my first set as a Christmas present the year of my ear incident. They changed my life at a time when I had hit bottom and could not tolerate much noise of any kind. I prefer the ones that cover the whole ear. They might be a bit larger, but they work better. Their tighter fit helps greatly in locking out noises. I have found the noise reduction is most effective for dampening background clamor in the low and medium frequency ranges. The shrieks of a crying baby are not softened by much, but it is a lot better than getting the full blast.

When buying noise-reducing earmuffs, it is important to check on the specifications. How much more peaceful will they make the world? Some are meant for home use and quieter settings, while others are designed for heavy-duty protection in noise-polluted environments, such as in the industry.

It seems that in our noisy world, the only things that stand between us and noise-induced hearing loss are awareness, good judgment, evasive action, and proper ear protection. Investing in our hearing is a wise long-term plan that will spare us unnecessary hardship in the future.

Antioxidants

Excessive noise hurts the sensitive cochlear hearing cells, both physically and metabolically. Overly intense sound stimulation revs up the cells' metabolism to the point of burnout and death. In the process of such metabolic overdrive, highly reactive chemicals known as "free radicals" are released. These are notorious for causing damage commonly referred to as "oxidative damage." In the cochlea, free radicals continue to be produced for some time, even after the noise insult has stopped, which leads to injury of yet more cells. If the abuse is repeated too often and for too long, the cumulative oxidative destruction eventually results in hearing loss.

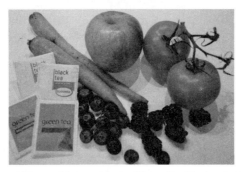

Many fruits, vegetables and tea contain healthy antioxidants. *photo: R.Hammond*

Chemicals that gobble up and neutralize free radicals are known as "antioxidants." These are nutrients found in green and black teas, fruits, berries, and many vegetables. Of course, pharmaceutical manufacturers also supply antioxidant pills and cocktails for easy consumption. Although the list of compounds is lengthy, we are mostly familiar with the vitamins C, E, and beta-carotene. In their quest to optimize our chances of avoiding NIHL, researchers continue to investigate different chemicals. The aim is to develop targeted antioxidant formulas that will serve as adjuncts to noise abatement strategies and ear protection.

The history of the antioxidant/free radical connection is rather interesting, and I shall digress for a moment in order to point out a few highlights. Antioxidants, which have become the darlings of TV health show hosts, rose to fame when scientists discovered that oxidative damage ravages the body in many ways. It causes aging and, most importantly, it can set off the chain of events that lead to cancer. These findings brought about an intense public health campaign aimed at preventing such noxious tissue injury. Among other recommendations, we were counseled to stay out of the sun and to quit smoking. We were also advised to increase our antioxidant intake by eating plenty of fruits and veggies and to boost a deficient diet with supplements.

Once it was recognized that noise-induced hearing loss is largely the result of free-radical damage, it made sense for scientists to explore how antioxidants could stem the harm. Although these compounds will *not fix or reverse* existing hearing loss, it is hoped that they might help prevent, or at least minimize, oxidative cochlear injury due to intense noise exposures.

Antioxidant vitamins, while the obvious frontrunners, are not the only agents whose possible hearing-protection capabilities are being investigated. They are only the obvious start. Researchers and manufacturers are busy identifying promising chemical candidates and testing them for safety and efficacy. Questions on dosages, drug interactions, side effects, contraindications, and timing must be answered. Dosages must be sufficiently high in order to produce helpful blood levels within the ears. Also, the timing of the doses must be right. How long before and/or after the noise exposure should the antioxidant product be taken for best results?

Although there is no shortage of antioxidant products on the market, so far the FDA has not approved any single compound or any combinations for the specific purpose of preventing noise-induced hearing loss (NIHL). Without that reassuring "clinically proven" label, how is the consumer to know or trust? I guess, as in so many situations, we are on our own.

Within reason, I believe in the overall antioxidant theory. As far as my hearing is concerned, I would certainly welcome any extra protection against NIHL that a specialized antioxidant product could offer. Yet I have trouble believing that I could fearlessly put my ears through prolonged and repeated decibel hurricanes just as long as I popped a pill. Antioxidants have their definite merits but they are not omnipotent. Although, at some point, the right antioxidant formula might provide us with an added safeguard and peace of mind, it cannot replace common sense and responsible behavior. For now, I keep carrying my earplugs—just in case.

Chapter 17
Ototoxic Substances

By definition, *ototoxicity* means that something is poisonous, or toxic, to the ears. During my first ENT clinic visit on the day of my sudden hearing loss, the ear specialists decided that chemical ototoxicity did not play a part in my predicament. There are, however, chemicals that can affect the ears adversely and, according to Dr. Todd, the possibility of this being a contributing factor to hearing loss or balance issues should always be considered.

Ototoxic damage concentrates on the inner ear—the cochlea and the vestibular system, involved with hearing and balance, respectively. The cochlear and/or the vestibular nerve(s) can also be affected. One hopes that such reactions will be temporary and disappear once the harmful substance is stopped. Yet any damage can be permanent and irreversible. Preventive strategies are best for dealing with the issue of ototoxicity. Yet it is not always possible to avoid medical treatments that involve possibly ototoxic agents. Also, a long list of contributing factors turn ototoxicity into a multifaceted medical challenge.

Some Symptoms

Not all ototoxic drugs have the same ear-damaging effects. Depending on the substance, ototoxic symptoms vary. Hearing loss, from mild to deafness, and/or dizziness and balance problems in response to chemical exposures, are not the only ototoxic effects. Unless it involves a drastic decline, an actual hearing loss is not that easy to detect. Obviously, if we do become aware of any change in hearing acuity, it is time to get help at once. Shifting or fluctuating hearing is more apparent and also must be reported without delay. Balance issues, dizziness, and lightheadedness, especially if accompanied by nausea, are understandably difficult to ignore. Tinnitus, however, a frequently reported ototoxic side effect, is a warning sign and might be an early indicator of hearing loss. For those who have tinnitus already, the tone may change or become louder. New or additional sounds might appear. People who never had tinnitus before might become aware of the appearance of the notorious buzzing, ringing, roaring or hissing sounds that can be steady or fade intermittently in and out. Hyperacusis—when everyday sounds seem way too loud—is another potential ototoxic effect. Auditory hallucinations—hearing things that are not there—have also been reported.

Whenever these or any other unsettling ear, hearing, and/ or equilibrium symptoms pop up in response to medications or supplements, patients should seek professional advice *at once.* They must report adverse inner-ear reactions that develop in response to a prescription drug *immediately* to the prescriber and insist on guidance for how to proceed. The health care provider who initiated the prescription decides if the dosage should be adjusted, if the medicine should be tapered off or stopped, or if it should be replaced with a different one. It is unwise to suddenly halt treatment, particularly without notifying the physician or other prescriber. Such practices could have unpleasant and dangerous consequences that go way beyond ear damage.

For over-the-counter medications or any other products intended for self-treatment, it makes sense to find information on ear-related side effects before purchasing the product(s). The pharmacist can help investigate or the doctor can offer an opinion. For those who do their own research, however, especially by relying on material found online, it is important to recognize when sites have a commercial or sales bias and offer little impartial information. When in doubt, it is best to consult the doctor or pharmacist.

Screening Prescriptions for Ototoxicity

Patients might do well to request an up-front ototoxicity search for any newly prescribed medication, especially if they have already hearing problems, tinnitus or balance issues. Besides doctors, other caregivers now have prescribing privileges and recommend over-the-counter products. Although they usually work under the guidance of a physician, it is nevertheless crucial for anyone who advises patients on drug treatments to be aware of possible ear-noxious effects.

Electronic databases with in-depth, current medication information are available to health professionals. Hospitals, pharmacies, and doctors' offices should be equipped with such new-age resources. Screening medications for ear-related side effects might reveal if there are any obvious reports on the drug itself or on drug interactions that could harm the inner ear and/or its nerves. Yet even with these high-tech systems, there are *no guarantees* that every minute detail for a specific medication will be listed. It is possible that ototoxic activity has never been reported for the agent in question or that the information we are looking for is simply not available.

Some Contributors to Ototoxicity

People who already have *existing* hearing and balance issues are considered to be more sensitive and at an increased risk for further problems due to ear-offensive chemicals. Some medications' ototoxic potential becomes more evident, depending on *the route of administration.* The intravenous (IV) route, which provides higher drug levels faster, can bring on ototoxic effects when oral therapy with the same drug at normal doses does not.

Ototoxicity also may be a function of *dose and length of treatment.* The higher the doses and the longer the exposure times, the higher the risk that a drug's ear-harming potential could become a threat. *Drug accumulation* also increases the chances for untoward reactions from possibly ototoxic medicines. Those with decreased liver and kidney

111

function are especially at risk, as their ability for properly breaking down and eliminating medications is hampered. Children whose liver and kidney functions are not yet fully developed and the elderly whose organs are slowing down must be monitored with special care.

Drug interactions can also contribute to ototoxicity. The chances for drug interactions increase with the number of medications used, especially if ear-endangering substances are involved. Drug interactions that lead to undesirable outcomes are caused by various mechanisms, such as medications reinforcing each other's effects, or the action of one drug slowing the metabolism of another. The potential for harmful drug interactions is increased further by patient *self-treatment* products, such as herbals, supplements, and over-the-counter medications. These compounds often are not reported to the primary care provider or to the pharmacy, and therefore do not figure on medication profiles. Any chemical, however, can contribute to drug interactions.

Then, there is the ever-present truth that we are all individuals with our own sensitivities. We all *react differently* to medications, and sometimes there is no good explanation why substances affect the ears of some people but not of others. In a field of ongoing research, scientists have found *genetic* links that predispose patients to the ear-toxic effects from some known offenders.

Overall, careful patient screening, responsible medication dosing, attention to drug interactions, cautious patient monitoring, and clear communication between patients and their health care providers contribute to keeping our ears at least reasonably safe.

Some Practical Points

Ototoxicity is a confusing issue for researchers, physicians, and patients alike. Ototoxic substances include environmental poisons, metals, herbals, supplements, substances of abuse, toxins such as snake or spider venoms, and of course, medications for both internal and external use. Depending on the source that one consults, the number of suspicious chemicals varies greatly. It is also confusing that not all references cite the same agents. It could be that authors differ in how they define "ototoxicity." Lists of suspected and known ototoxic agents are readily available, although they might not be current. I included some sources in the reference section for this chapter. Instead of focusing on the long litany of substances, I will touch on a few practical aspects of this baffling topic.

As I mentioned earlier, many factors can aggravate or contribute to a medication's ototoxic potential. The fact that a chemical or drug has been placed on a watch list does not necessarily mean that it will be harmful to everyone, to the same degree, in the same way, all of the time. We are forewarned of possible problems, however, once a drug's ear-harmful effects are reported. Although doctors generally try to find non-ototoxic alternatives, there are instances when there are few other choices. This is why it is important to address any ear-concerns with the physician ahead of time and to understand why treatment with a potentially ototoxic medicine is necessary.

When it comes to medications, some of the worst offenders are well known. Although not all cancer *chemotherapy* drugs are ototoxic, doctors keep a watchful eye on a select number that are recognized for their ear-noxious action. All chemotherapy agents, however, are administered under strict specialist supervision. The professionals who work with these drugs are aware of the ototoxic issue and monitor and counsel the patient appropriately. Unfortunately, cancer treatment is one of those situations where alternative options might be limited, as the drugs must be chosen based on their cancer-fighting activities.

Another group of medications with known ototoxic potential are the antibiotics known as *aminoglycosides*. It has been found that a genetic predisposition can make people sensitive to the ear-damaging effects of these drugs. Administered by injection in clinical settings, pharmacists are often entrusted with the dosing of at least two of the better-known members of this family namely, gentamicin and tobramycin. Careful dosing and meticulous patient monitoring can greatly reduce, if not eliminate, their ototoxic impact. Alone or in combination with other medications, aminoglycoside products are also available for treating certain eye, ear, and skin infections. The guidelines for prescribing aminoglycoside-containing *ear drops* caution against using them if the eardrum is damaged or perforated.

Ads for medicines used to treat erectile dysfunction (ED) now mention that hearing loss can be a side effect of these agents. The hearing decline can be sudden or rapid and may be accompanied by tinnitus and/or dizziness.

As patients, we are most often at risk when we purchase products for *self-treatment* and make unassisted decisions on our own behalf. The aminoglycoside neomycin is a common ingredient in over-the-counter creams and ointments for treating skin infections. Although these products are meant to be applied lightly, short-term to *small* cuts and scrapes, people often use them on larger, open wounds for lengthy periods of time. Such action might well allow for the absorption of a sufficient amount of drug to cause ototoxicity concerns, especially in already predisposed people. Therefore, caution is the word. We must read and follow the instructions exactly. We must also remember that large, open wounds are best cleaned and treated professionally as are small wounds that refuse to heal.

Especially if they are taken at high doses for long periods of time, popular over-the-counter pain relievers, such as aspirin and nonsteroidal anti-inflammatory drugs (NSAIDs) are mentioned for their potential to cause tinnitus and even hearing loss. It came as a surprise when even acetaminophen (Tylenol) was implicated in causing hearing damage. This is why it is important to discuss nagging pain issues with the doctor and to ask the advice of the pharmacist when purchasing products for self-care.

Watching Out for Ourselves

Due to the often spotty information and the many uncertainties that surround the issue of ototoxicity, there are no guarantees that our inner ears and their nerves will be safe on all counts from medications and other health products. We can take some actions, however, that will keep us out of harm's way.

While it is unnecessary to memorize the names of all known or suspected ototoxic substances, it is important for us to be aware that many chemicals can indeed cause ear damage. We are also well served if we know at least the most important telltale symptoms of drug-induced ear issues. Most of all, good communication with doctors and pharmacists is of the utmost importance. It falls on us to inform all of our health care specialists—physicians, pharmacists, dentists, eye doctors, audiologists, and therapists—about our hearing, balance, and other ear problems.

We also must ask prescribers about ear-compromising effects of medications that are ordered for us—and do so *before* we leave the clinic. Maybe it is just me, but once I leave the physician's office, it almost takes a federal decree for me to reconnect, should I have any extra questions. If the pharmacy determines later on that a particular prescribed drug raises concerns, it becomes much more difficult to address these issues. Treatment is on hold while the problem is resolved through telephone or email tag.

Never underestimate the value of a healthy dose of curiosity; there is nothing wrong with being inquisitive. A lot more information is available to patients now than there ever used to be. It is to our benefit to learn as much as we can about our medications, including their ototoxic potential.

Pharmacists are always good information sources, especially if we are choosing over-the-counter products. For any new prescriptions, it pays to accept the pharmacist's counseling that is offered when picking up our medications. This gives us one more opportunity to double-check on drug interactions and on possible ear-toxic effects.

We also should make it a rule to read all the information that is included with a prescription or over-the-counter medicine. Those with truly inquiring minds might make use of their computer to check on a medication or supplement at a reputable website. Most of all, we *must notify the physician at once* if we experience ototoxic side effects, such as tinnitus, balance issues, dizziness, hearing loss, hearing downshifts or hearing fluctuations in response to a medication.

FDA MedWatch: Let's Share

As a contribution to mankind, should we report a suspected ototoxic medication to the Food and Drug Administration (FDA)? Absolutely! Clinical studies run before a drug is released onto the market certainly provide a lot of important information. Yet they only last for a specified time and involve limited populations of test subjects. Once the drug becomes available to all of us, however, the true trial begins. We become the ultimate testing ground, with our individual genetic make-ups, sensitivities, and health conditions. I believe that any post-marketing information that health providers and the public can supply is most important for learning the good, the bad, and the ugly details about medications.

Over the years, scores of medications have appeared—and then disappeared because of supplemental issues that did not raise an eyebrow during the pre-marketing phases. The FDA has a safety and adverse events reporting program called MedWatch that can be accessed online at www.fda.gov/medwatch. It is through this program that post-marketing drug information reaches the government. Reports on problem-causing drugs can be completed directly online. As an alternative, a printout of the online form can be used for a mail-in paper-and-pencil report. If evidence shows that there might be a concern with a certain medication, the FDA will take the necessary steps to contact manufacturers and alert prescribers. By sharing their experience, patients' efforts could well bring a drug's ototoxic potential under much-needed scrutiny.

Chapter 18
The MRI

MRI stands for "magnetic resonance imaging." These are wonderfully complicated, non-invasive scans that do not expose us to any radiation. An MRI looks inside the body by means of magnetic field and radio wave energy. The pictures are digital, and their resolution can be enhanced by the administration of intravenous contrast material.

Prior to my ear event, I had never had an MRI, and I was kind of curious how this would proceed. In the afternoon of Day 2, I got ready for the test with the help of Nurse Lisa.

In my years of working in hospitals, I learned that the narrow "tube" could trigger claustrophobia and anxiety attacks in those who hate confined spaces. I knew that a fair share of people became agitated during the procedure and wanted out of the pipe, now. I also knew that I could be sedated or put to sleep, if necessary, in order to make it through the test. Yet I was to learn a lot more firsthand. My being moderately claustrophobic turned out not to be my major MRI issue.

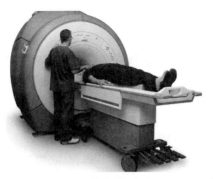

Ready for the MRI. It will be loud. Get ear protection.
photo: (c) jgroup www.fotosearch.com

119

As I mentioned earlier in the story, before my scan began, the MRI tech asked me if I wanted to listen to music during the test. This was the best offer I had had all day, and I gladly accepted. An assistant gave me a set of headphones and mentioned that they would "reduce noise." At the moment I did not understand why that would be important, but I would be enlightened soon.

While I tried to relax inside the scanner, the racket began. BRRR ... BRRR—there were bone-jarring noises right around my head. Nobody had warned me about this. I tested the audio, asking what this was all about. I was told that the testing parts of the machine had to be rotated, adjusted, and aligned. The noise was simply the "nature of the beast." Another BRRR and then BAM, BAM, BAM—the actual scan was now in progress. The explanation that these were "gradient coil vibration noises" did not help, although it was an interesting tech tidbit. Trapped within this sound nightmare, I felt like being at a rock concert with the head stuck inside the bass drum. *Oh, please, do not kill off my good ear!* I thought.

The flimsy headphones that were supposed to help dampen the ruckus did not fit tightly enough. No one checked their position on my ears, and now I could not move in order to adjust them. I would have asked for additional earplugs, had I only known. Although the dreadful din just about got the best of me, in the end, it was all worth it. The "beast" did not unearth any worrisome details, such as growths, tumors, inner ear fluid leaks, bone fissures, or signs of stroke.

As MRI scanners have become more powerful, the noise inside the tubes has increased to levels that fall well within the danger zone of 100 decibels and more. Researchers are seriously concerned by the MRI clatter, and fortunately, many great ideas have been put forth to alleviate the noise. Active noise-control systems are aimed at reducing the sound field at ear level. Engineers also have worked on decreasing disruptive whirlwind currents in various parts of the machine, as well as stabilizing and supporting the noisy coils while enclosing them in vacuum chambers. Such endeavors all promise to greatly reduce the MRI noise level.

The new "open" MRI scanners that allow patients to sit down or even stand are less claustrophobic and are said to produce less knocking noise than the standard tube-edition. I suppose that this amounts to a gentler BRRR, BRRR and BAM, BAM. There is even talk about "silent" MRI technology in the future, which would do away with noisy gradient coils. What a relief that will be.

As far as noise exposures are concerned, I prefer to err on the side of safety—my hearing loss has taught me that. If I ever must submit to another MRI scan, I will insist on *maximum ear protection*. Now that I am aware, I will adjust the fit of the headphones and request additional earplugs. Measurements have shown that even with the standard MRI technology, correctly inserted earplugs, combined with well-fitting earmuffs, can push the ear-level clamor down into the acceptable decibel range.

CHAPTER 19
Tumors

After the MRI was done, the orderly brought me back to the station. Nurse Lisa felt that I had been through enough for one day and recommended that I should rest for a while. How could I possibly rest when the word "tumor" seemed to be written everywhere? I could think of all sorts of scenarios, none of them in my favor.

Of course, any growth within the head that is capable of putting pressure on the eighth cranial nerve could cause hearing loss and/or balance problems. Also known as the vestibulo-cochlear nerve, this nerve serves the inner ear. It is made of two separate branches, the cochlear nerve and the vestibular nerve. The cochlear nerve carries hearing impulses to the brain, while the vestibular nerve informs the brain on balance.

During my ENT clinic visit, Dr. Todd had mentioned that the specific tumors that the MRI would hunt for were *vestibular schwannomas,* or *acoustic neuromas.* These are benign growths that can form on the eighth cranial nerve. They favor the vestibular portion over the cochlear portion and are usually unilateral, which means that they affect only one side.

Nerves are basically electrical wires, and just like electrical wires they are insulated in order to protect them from damage and from "shorting out." The special insulating and supporting cells that wrap around the vestibular and cochlear nerve trunks are called the *Schwann cells.* An overproduction of these cells leads to the formation of benign clumps, or tumors, that follow different growth patterns. Usually, they are slow growing, although some can develop relatively quickly.

When the clumps are tiny, there might not be any symptoms, but as they develop and increase in size, they can become worrisome. Gradually, they start to press against the balance and/or hearing nerves, which results in dizziness and equilibrium disturbances, as well as one-sided hearing loss and tinnitus. Pressure on adjacent nerves that serve the face and jaw may lead to facial numbness and weakness. Once they are large enough to put pressure on actual brain structures, vestibular schwannomas can become life-threatening. Although benign, these expanding tumors can cause major havoc, as the skull is a bony box, and there is not much room for spreading out.

I had inquired earlier which action the doctors would take, should such a schwannoma be found. I was told that this would depend on the size of the growth, its location, and on how much damage had already been done. We could just watch it; remove it surgically, the old-fashioned way; or apply a type of radiation treatment known as "radiosurgery." Brain radiosurgery involves high doses of radiation that are delivered to the growth with pinpoint accuracy by a machine referred to as "Gamma Knife," although no cutting is involved in the procedure. Dr. Leonard, the voice of experience, stated at the time that "just watching it" was not an option. If any tumor showed up, it would be dealt with, the earlier the better.

After the MRI, I lay in bed, exhausted but unable to sleep. Life passed in front of me in slow motion—thanks to all the medication concoctions that had been administered to me throughout the day. In my listless mind, I simply could not imagine that someone would dig around in my ear or brain or that I would be irradiated until I glowed in the dark. It ended up being a long night. The following morning, Dr. Todd brought me the good news that no tumors had been found.

Chapter 20
Equilibrium and Balance:
Ears, Eyes, and Body Sensors

On that infamous day of my ear attack, cochlear damage brought me hearing loss and many other challenges. Vestibular system damage threw me terribly off-kilter. A few hours after my hearing took a nosedive, I was unable to stand up, walk, or move my head in any direction. Any little wiggle at once brought on a violent, super-nausea-inducing spin known as vertigo. The world whirled at lightning speed. The hearing loss was traumatic and upsetting, but ultimately the balance and vertigo issues brought me to the decision that I was in acute distress and needed medical help.

The Equilibrium Tripod
In order to keep us balanced, the brain gets feedback from the vestibular system of our *inner ears*, from the *eyes*, and from *proprioceptors,* which are sensors located in the muscles, tendons, and joints. One might think of the "equilibrium tripod." By working as a team, these three entities continuously inform the brain about our equilibrium status. Should we be thrown off balance, the "righting reflex" helps to get us centered again.

Actually, our moving about on two legs while holding ourselves upright puts the balance mechanisms seriously to the test. Most of the time, we are in a state of impending disequilibrium and at risk for falls. In physics terms, our center of gravity is high. A high center of gravity means that the object, in this case the human body, is unstable and tends to tip over easily. Unless all of our balance processes are well-tuned, gravity becomes our enemy. The equilibrium mechanisms are phenomenally complex. Plenty of minute details on how they work together and communicate with one another still remain mysteries. Until my balance tripod lost a leg or two, I had never given much thought to everything that was involved in keeping me from ending up in a body cast.

Under normal circumstances, maintaining one's balance is an ongoing day-and-night process of which we are not even aware. But I got my wake-up call, and now I have to think before I turn or make sudden moves. Ever since I wound up crawling on all fours, I watch figure skating with a different appreciation. As the skater hurls himself into space to land that quad, I am awed by the complexities of our balance feedback systems.

Balance and the Ears: the Vestibular System

The inner ear is a very small, congested place. It houses the sensing organs for hearing and balance—the cochlea, in charge of hearing, and the vestibular system, in charge of balance.

The vestibular system is made up of five sensor organs: three semicircular ducts located in the bony semicircular canals and two otoliths organs, or ear-rock bodies, the utricle and saccule, which are located in an area called the vestibule. As body and head movements involve all sorts of positions, speeds, and directions, the five structures work together in an effort to maintain balance.

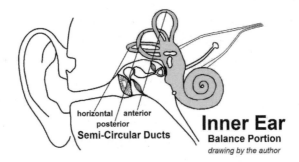

horizontal / anterior
posterior
Semi-Circular Ducts

Inner Ear
Balance Portion
drawing by the author

126

The semicircular ducts are roughly at right angles to one another, which means that each one points in a different direction—forward, backward, and sideways. The ducts are filled with endolymph fluid. At its base, each duct is outfitted with tufts of special *motion* sensor cells that detect orientation and speed of movements, as the head turns and rotates in all directions. Let's just say that the semicircular structures get a workout, as the skater spins while delivering that elegant precision pirouette. As our head moves about, so does the endolymph in the appropriate duct. Endolymph movement stimulates the sensor cells, which generate electrical impulses that are relayed to the brain by the vestibular nerve.

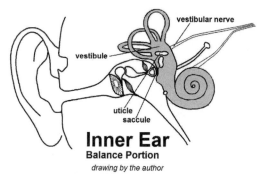

Inner Ear
Balance Portion
drawing by the author

The otoliths organs, the utricle and the saccule, contain *gravity* sensor cells that monitor the head's *position* at rest. They also report on linear, straight-line head movements, such as leaning forward or backward or going from a lying to a sitting position. The tips of the otolith sensor hair cells are lodged in a gooey, gelatin-like substance into which ear rocks, or otoconia, are embedded. If our head moves in a straight line or if its position changes, the otoconia slide or drag across the sticky mass, thereby stimulating the tips of the sensor cells beneath. In response, the cells generate electrical impulses that travel to the brain via the vestibular nerve. The utricle is located close to the openings of the semicircular ducts. The saccule is positioned closer to the cochlea.

127

The utricle detects when the head is tilted forward, backward, or sideways. If I sit looking down while reading a book, or if I stand still and gaze up at the stars, the utricle informs the brain on my head's position in relation to gravity. The saccule knows when the head is in a vertical or upright position. If I sit still, looking straight ahead as I watch a movie, the saccule becomes my brain's informant.

Occasionally, otoconia break loose from the *utricle* and wander into one of the semicircular ducts. Now these crystals float into the canal's endolymph where they wind up stimulating the motion-sensing cells. This unleashes awful dizziness and unsteadiness episodes. The action of the wayward otoconia is the basis for benign paroxismal positional vertigo (BPPV).

Why these ear rocks break away from their base is often not known and in that case the cause for BPPV is said to be "idiopathic," which means "of unknown cause." However, head injury, weakening or degeneration of vestibular structures due to advancing age, infections, and other disorders that attack the inner ear may have harmed the utricle. Typically, symptoms are brought on by a change in head position with respect to gravity. People who are affected by this condition usually know which head movements will get them into trouble.

Rolling over in bed or lying flat on one's back for lengthy periods can be enough to bring on a BPPV attack. A backward tilt of the head, however, seems to be one of the more notorious triggers. One of my coworkers was unable to look upward when reaching for items in her cabinets. If no one was around to lend a helping hand, she would climb on a stool to keep her head straight. The nausea that accompanies BBPV usually convinces patients to seek medical help. As we have already seen, dizziness and balance symptoms can be associated with many different issues, such as a viral infection, a vestibular Schwannoma, a stroke, Ménière's disease, and so on. Because there are so many other conditions that could be mistaken for BPPV, it is important to see a doctor who has experience with these problems for a proper diagnosis and testing.

Once it is determined that BPPV is indeed the culprit, the main treatment goal is to coax the errant ear rocks out of the semicircular canal and back into a place within the vestibule where they do not cause havoc. By applying a series of well-orchestrated body positions and head movements, the doctor can treat BPPV in the emergency room or in the office. One of the commonly used sequences is called the *Epley maneuver.* Named after its inventor Dr. John Epley, it is also known as the "canalith repositioning procedure" (CRP). After the treatment, the patient is discharged with specific instructions for follow-up. For patients who have been formally diagnosed and who have experience with BPPV, a home version of the Epley maneuver is available. Medication can be prescribed for nausea control.

Balance and the Eyes

Our vision orients us in space and thereby plays an important part in helping us maintain our balance. The eyes give feedback to the brain regarding the body's position and movement in the surrounding world. Do we move, or do things around us move? Once we close our eyes, it is actually hard to stay balanced without swaying.

As we move and as our heads move, however, objects and the world around us are kept in focus, thanks to the vestibular-ocular reflex (VOR). This reflex keeps the eyes steady and aligned as the head moves. It is the result of highly sophisticated nerve connections between the inner-ear balance system and the muscles that control the eyes. In order to keep our equilibrium, the direct interaction between eyes and inner ears is very much needed.

I have often wondered if a confused VOR was to blame for my watering eyes and for my not being able to see "fast enough," especially during the initial throes of my ear debacle. Everything seemed to be off—and maybe it was.

Balance and the Body Sensors

Designated areas of the brain also receive information from special sensors located throughout the body in muscles, joints, and tendons. Known as "proprioceptors," they specialize in monitoring joint angles as well as tissue tension and pressure. As we Jazzercise, how do our legs move in comparison to our arms or torso? Do we walk, or do we run? Are we standing or sitting down? The brain knows, because the proprioceptors help set the record straight.

A lot of counterbalancing must be done for us not to fall over, especially under challenging circumstances. A network of nervous connections between the vestibular system and the spinal cord accounts for yet another collection of reflexes called the vestibulospinal reflex (VSR). It helps to steady the body by adjusting posture and muscle tone. The VSR usually refers to reflex action involving muscles *below* the neck and does not include another most important inner-ear/muscle reflex, known as the vestibulocollic reflex (VCR). The VCR concerns itself with the neck muscles that stabilize the head.

Together with a series of other reflexes, all of these systems act as a team, every second of our lives, whether we are asleep or awake, in order to integrate any of our movements, no matter how insignificant. The ears, eyes, and body sensors do such a good job orchestrating their every action that we are hardly ever aware of the miracle of balance—until suddenly, one tiny thing goes wrong. I am still amazed by how much I took this for granted all of these years.

Dizziness and Imbalance: Are the Ears Always to Blame?

I have days when my balance is threatened because I feel lightheaded and off-kilter. I am aware that my VOR and VSR are no longer what they used to be, and I know why. Some time ago, my inner ear got whacked, and the delicate balance system (and maybe its nerve) took a hit. Many people, however, do not know why they are plagued by feelings of dizziness, lightheadedness, or generalized disequilibrium that put serious limitations on their lives and may lead to falls and injuries.

Often the reason for feeling faint or wobbly is not due to vestibular damage. A multitude of other causes can produce some of the same symptoms. For instance, other than an inner ear problem, feeling woozy and unsteady might be related to a medication or supplement side effect, a drug interaction, a heart issue, blocked arteries that restrict blood flow to the head and heart, blood pressure problems, a stroke, a blood disorder like anemia, blood sugar fluctuations, dehydration, a brain tumor, an electrolyte imbalance, failing vision, badly adjusted eyeglasses, anxiety, and neurological concerns, to name a few.

I have worked all of my life in hospitals. A major reason why people come to the emergency room is dizziness and subsequent nausea and/or injuries due to falls. Many report having had symptoms for some time. I believe that anyone who is pestered by persistent feelings of dizziness, lightheadedness or unsteadiness needs a medical workup in order to find the cause and get a diagnosis. It might have nothing to do with the ears. Maybe there is another obvious explanation. Maybe something can be fixed. At any rate, it is important to follow up.

Chapter 21
Regaining Balance

By the time of my discharge from the hospital, I was able to shuffle around the room—at least it was progress. I went home with the strict warning that I had to work on my equilibrium situation. The goal was to teach the brain how to compensate for my vestibular deficit. There were various ways to tackle the challenge.

Equilibrium Training at Home

As I had improved somewhat and was able to count on the help of my husband, my doctors believed that I could give balance rehabilitation a try at home. Dr. Leonard told me, though, that I would be referred at once, should I need the expertise of a specially trained therapist. The discharge nurse said she was confident that a "flexible spring chicken" like me could manage. Honestly, I felt more like a stiff old hen. Earlier, during my stopover at the doctor's office, I already had been handed a fistful of lists with a variety of safety instructions and equilibrium exercises. The Valium that was prescribed upon discharge was to help my confused and stressed vestibular system settle down.

Although I was able to walk somewhat independently, my eye/hand coordination and depth perception were way off. There are plenty of reminders around the house that I dropped and nicked a lot of stuff in those days, and then there were continuous spills. Today, my VOR is still sort of shaky now and then, but I am doing a lot better.

At the outset, I needed firm assistance, which was very frustrating. I had to relearn how to stand up straight without stooping or tilting, walk in a straight line without weaving all over, negotiate the stairs without missing steps, move my head gently in all directions without swaying, fix my gaze, move my eyes, and so on. My equilibrium "tripod" was seriously compromised.

The in-home training sessions took a lot of patience and self-indoctrination: read the drill instructions, internalize them, concentrate, do the task. I felt like I was in some balance boot camp. I never concentrated so hard on anything in my life as I did at that point on just walking—yet another reminder that life had indeed changed. After a while, I did relatively well inside the house: the next step was to go for an afternoon walk. Once I stepped outside, the challenges began. Conflicting noises that were way too loud, scattering sound, increases in tinnitus, and my lopsided hearing created problems and did not help my equilibrium one bit. My eyes watered, and my vision was blurry. There was too much light, too much noise—a total sensory overload. The first outings were short, but I was proud of myself that I ventured into a world that had turned into a somewhat hostile place.

Over time, gradually, I regained some sense of normalcy. Walks in the neighborhood became longer. My husband had to hang on to me—and he still does—because of my tendency to pull to the side and head for the shrubs. Never did we hold hands more firmly and consistently than on those walks. I still weave and probably always will, yet progress has been made. Now, I am able to go out by myself. I can also drive to the grocery store and make short trips to the mall. I have become less aware of my being out of balance, but the reminders are never far away.

Professional Equilibrium Training

For many people, an at-home exercise program like mine is not appropriate or not enough to help. Had I not been able to manage, I would not have hesitated to seek the help and advice of a therapist trained in *Vestibular Rehabilitation Therapy (VRT)*. VRT helps teach the brain how to coordinate information from the vestibular system. Muscle-strengthening exercises might also be needed. Although there are a variety of programs that offer balance retraining, I think it is best to ask the physician or audiologist for a referral to a reliable clinic. Therapists need to be properly trained in the specific techniques that make up VRT. Based on the patient's diagnosis and medical findings, the practitioner evaluates the severity of the case and takes into consideration the patient's age, lifestyle, and physical ability, among other points. An exercise program is then designed that serves the individual's needs.

In a couple of sessions a week, for four to six weeks, clients are shown routine exercises for daily living and practice more challenging tasks, such as following moving objects with the eyes, climbing stairs, walking on uneven or rough terrain, and transitioning from bare floor to carpeting. They also learn how and when to use assistive devices, such as canes or walkers. Participants work under the guidance and supervision of a therapist. Many appreciate the reassurance and encouragement of a professional presence.

I have met quite a few people who feel that VRT helped them enormously, not only physically but also emotionally. A lady told me that the therapy helped her regain her self-confidence, which was seriously lacking. When she started on the program, she only knew her limits—what she could *not* do. She was amazed to learn that there were ways around those limits and how much she actually *could do.*

No matter what the approach, after a while, the newly learned equilibrium strategies work themselves into daily life. Still, there are those moments when we forget that we should not whip around so fast or sprint for the bus. Exercises by themselves do not cure vestibular disorders or prevent falls. They teach us, however, how to compensate for our shortcomings and how to anticipate and avoid problem situations. That is a big step in the right direction.

***

That Floating Feeling

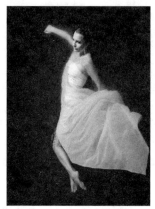

Those with vestibular issues can feel like they are floating on air.
photo: (c) Julenochek www.fotosearch.com

I guess that I will never know what made me "float." My equilibrium would become seriously challenged in wide open-space areas, such as shopping malls or hotel lobbies with large central halls or vaulted atria; churches with arched, high ceilings; or huge stores. There seemed to be a subliminal hum in the air.

It was only a matter of time, after I stepped into such a place, before I became extremely tired and maybe a touch spacey. It was as if someone lifted me out of my shoes. I felt ten pounds lighter—wow, if that had only been true! I wobbled about almost aimlessly, stepping as if I were walking on cotton balls. After a while, all I could think of was to get out of there. I came to refer to this feeling as "the big-hall effect." Earplugs helped quite a bit but it took me a while to discover that. I learned to identify "big halls" that were likely to cause me grief. I planned my trips, stuck to shopping lists, and spent as little time there as possible.

Yet I wondered why I was fine in some places but not in others. My descriptions and questions drew many a raised eyebrow and incredulous look from medical specialists. One audiologist nodded her head in agreement but did not offer an explanation. Eventually, I quit asking. I had not expected any earth-shattering revelations, but it bugged me that no one could help me even work out a theory that could make sense.

Subsequently, I found references that indicated that people with vestibular problems often complain of a false sense of motion and of "floating" sensations. It felt good to know that I was not the only one who had ever experienced this. I was not some deranged person with an overly active imagination after all.

Once I began to attend support groups, I raised the issue of the floating feeling in one of our meetings. Amazingly, there were quite a few people who knew immediately what I meant by the "big-hall effect." All had vestibular issues, and none of them had ever gotten an explanation for the strange episodes. Terms such as "becoming disconnected in large spaces," "stumbling around in a big barn," "feeling hollow and eerily light," "my feet don't touch the ground" were only some of the ways that the sensation was described.

I do not know why or when it stopped happening, but I rarely ever "float" anymore. Maybe the vestibular system has stabilized itself somewhat? Although I still become rather quickly exhausted in large-hall settings, I go grocery shopping without floating. I have wandered for hours at the airport, waiting for my plane, without floating before flying. I survived an overseas trip that involved spending time in many huge spaces. To this day, though, I am still weary of big halls and tend not to linger. I do not want to challenge my good fortune. I am glad that the issue *seems* to have resolved itself. The feeling is mostly gone—and I hope that it stays that way.

Chapter 22
Sudden Sensorineural Hearing Loss (SSHL)

On the day of my discharge from the hospital, the physician who filled in for Dr. Leonard introduced me briefly to the notion of sudden sensorineural hearing loss (SSHL)—my tentative diagnosis. Although it can happen to younger people, the incidence increases as we reach our mid-forties to mid-fifties. Men and women are equally affected.

I pointed out earlier that the word "sensori" refers to the snail-like hearing organ, the cochlea, and its hearing cells. The word "neural" refers to the cochlear nerve that transfers information from the cochlea to the brainstem and/or other nervous pathways involved with hearing. In SSHL, damage to any one or more of these structures can result in a rapid hearing decline. In addition to the hearing loss, roughly 50 percent of patients also have symptoms of vestibular system involvement, which translate into vertigo, nausea, and balance problems. I had it all.

Criteria that define SSHL state that this is a hearing loss of greater than 30 dB over three consecutive pure-tone test frequencies. The decline proceeds fast, over no more than three days. Usually, only one ear is involved. Ear "fullness" is a common complaint, and the majority of patients experience tinnitus in the affected ear.

It took me all of four hours before I was as deaf as a post in my left ear, which felt as if it were stuffed with cotton balls. Unrelenting buzzing started on the day after this dramatic event, and it has not stopped for one minute since.

SSHL: A Medical Emergency

In spite of being quite worried, as my hearing faded away, I did not feel any urgency over going immediately to the hospital. After all, I did not have any pain or a fever. I did decide to see the physician the following day, but other than that, I went home and failed to take action. Ultimately, vertigo and severe nausea convinced me to go for help. Although many patients may regain hearing spontaneously, without any treatment, SSHL is a warning that something is seriously wrong. The condition is mostly considered as a *symptom* of some underlying condition. The professional literature commonly refers to SSHL as a *medical emergency*. It is important to seek medical help at once to find out what the underlying process might be or what it is not.

Although there are many possible causes for SSHL, a single, definitive answer often cannot be pinpointed, in spite of extensive testing; this is frustrating for both the patient and the doctor. If no clear reason is found, the condition is labeled as being "idiopathic" in nature, which means that the "cause is unknown." Only 10 to 15 percent of those affected with SSHL ever learn what caused their predicament.

After I wrote an article for a local paper describing my adventure, I received calls from various people who had experienced hearing loss symptoms very similar to mine. One lady woke up one morning to find that one of her ears had gone almost deaf overnight. After a weeklong wait for a doctor's appointment, she was treated for an ear infection, which she felt did not help her. At the time we talked, she had made little progress. Another woman had a milder sudden loss. She never went to the doctor but reported that her hearing improved quite a bit on its own, which is not unusual. Both women mentioned that wondering about what might have provoked their symptoms had caused them quite a bit of worry.

The Long List of Possible Causes

A widely held belief is that a good portion of SSHL cases are due to some sort of viral infection. Adenoviruses that cause respiratory infections, cytomegalovirus (CMV), and influenza viruses all figure on the lengthy list of possible offenders. The *herpes simplex type 1* virus (HSV-1), however, has emerged as the number one suspect. We know it commonly as the cold sore or fever blister virus, even though it can also cause encephalitis and serious infections of the skin and eyes.

There are over a hundred possible reasons why people lose their hearing suddenly. After all the test results were in, a virus still was the most plausible culprit for my woes. It had been determined that ototoxic substance side effects were not at play. An electrocardiogram (EKG), done in the emergency room, excluded a heart condition. The MRI and blood tests eliminated other common causes, such as physical ear and head damage, ear growths and tumors, autoimmune disease, stroke, syphilis, and blood disorders. As these are all rather worrisome scenarios, it was comforting to know that they did *not* contribute to my condition. On my first follow-up visit, Dr. Leonard supported Dr. Todd's "perfect ear storm theory," which related my predicament to a combination of viral infection, excessive noise exposure, and a possible stress-induced blood vessel spasm. The likelihood, however, that my ear event might have been a first attack of Ménière's disease remained an option for some time.

SSHL: Drug Treatment

Although the cause is often unknown, it is still accepted that SSHL could be the result of damage brought on by one or more ear-noxious processes that might not be immediately obvious or detectable. Until tests determine the underlying cause or causes, drug treatment for SSHL is speculative. Symptoms are managed and *suspected* contributing conditions are addressed in ways that are dictated largely by the doctor's practical experience with the condition.

As I related earlier, my medication regimen included agents meant to stem the damage related to a possible viral origin and/or immune component. The drugs used to treat me, however, do not represent the only options and choices available for treating a patient with my symptoms and suspected diagnosis. They were simply the medicines that my doctors decided were the most appropriate in my case.

Currently, corticosteroids, given orally or by direct injection into the ear, are the only medications considered to be helpful to some degree in some cases. Although they might not work for everyone, many physicians believe that patients should be offered the potential benefit of these agents as soon as possible, unless their health condition does not allow for it.

Medication treatment for SSHL, however, can also stir up controversy. As people often recover on their own or regain at least some hearing without medical intervention, this might suggest that no treatment is indicated. There are those who would argue that the use of medications is irrational at best, as some studies report no difference between patients who were treated with various drug regimens and those who were not. Although there might not be any obvious reasons for most SSHL cases, something alarming obviously happened. Doctors are generally not inclined to take a wait-and-see attitude with patients who present with SSHL and rely on their best hunches to help the patient.

I was certainly glad that my physician team did *not* opt for "doing nothing." If they had sent me home, hoping for a spontaneous recovery, it would have been emotionally devastating to me. I would wonder for the rest of my life what difference drug treatment could have made. The prednisone/antiviral combination that had been started in the hospital made great sense to me. I felt I only would gain from the experiment. In retrospect, it was a rough road, but I am glad that I stayed the course. Getting back some notion of sound within thirty-six hours of such a massive hearing loss was certainly most uplifting. Detractors might suggest that I recovered spontaneously, but I believe that support from my medications gave me a head start on the way to recovery.

Chapter 23
Ménière's Disease

The discharge physician certainly rattled my cage when he mentioned Ménière's disease once more as a possible cause for my predicament. I did not know any specific details, other than that vertigo could make people with this inner ear disorder quite ill. Having just experienced a dizziness episode where my head felt as if it was in a salad spinner, the Ménière's option sounded ominous, and I feared the worst. For people with inner ear and vertigo symptoms, Ménière's disease figures prominently on the list of possible causes. After an intense medical search does not reveal any obvious other reasons for the patient's complaints, a diagnosis of Ménière's disease is often put forth.

The condition was first described in 1861 by the French ear specialist Prosper Ménière. In the year before his death, he published his observations on the condition that now bears his name. He described the symptoms and also identified the inner ear as the origin of the disorder, which proved to be true.

Ménière's Disease: Classic and Atypical

Classic Ménière's disease is a non-fatal, chronic, and progressive condition that involves the entire inner ear—the cochlea as well as the balance structures. Usually, one ear is affected, but within years, both ears can become involved. As time goes on, most people notice a progressive, low-frequency hearing loss in the target ear and may be bothered by lingering equilibrium problems. The classic version of the disorder is characterized by *four symptoms* that are all described as episodic and fluctuating: hearing loss, vertigo, tinnitus, and ear fullness. Episodes that are highlighted by a crescendo of these four symptoms are referred to as "attacks," which can range from mild to incapacitating.

Just to complicate the picture, there are two subcategories to classic Ménière's disease. They are characterized by only three of the above telltale signs and are therefore considered "atypical." *Cochlear* Ménière's disease has all the episodic, fluctuating symptoms *except* vertigo. *Vestibular* Ménière's disease has all the episodic, fluctuating symptoms *except* hearing loss. Over time, an atypical Ménière's variant can morph into the classic form, complete with all four symptoms.

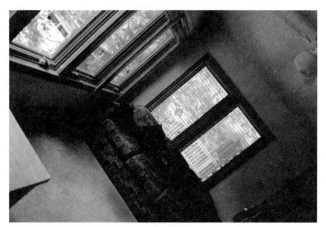

During an attack, some people describe a feeling that the world is on its side.
Sudden vertigo or "spinning rooms" can often precede Meniere's attacks.
photo: R.Hammond

Symptoms and Attacks

I attend a support group that serves mostly Ménière's disease and tinnitus patients. I have been told that Ménière's symptoms can pop up at any time. They come and go and vary in duration and intensity. Quite a few people report that they are never quite symptom-free. There are good days, not-so-good days, bad days, and really bad days. "Really bad days" are characterized by spinning attacks that can hit without much warning.

Attacks themselves also vary in severity and are universally described as scary and debilitating. They might be brief surges of symptoms, or they may last for hours. They are punctuated by the classic signs of hearing downshift, tinnitus that is often described as roaring, ear fullness, and dizziness that usually leads to nausea and vomiting. There is no way of predicting the frequency of the attacks. They may be separated by extended periods of time—weeks, months, or maybe years—yet they can also come in clusters with several attacks happening at close intervals. Every case and every incident is different.

Some of the more unsettling Ménière's disease accounts relate to sudden events known as "*drop attacks.*" These can lead to grave physical injury. I have heard such attacks described in two ways. Some people tell of feeling abruptly off balance, as if they were leaning or slumping over, although they are perfectly upright. Instinctively, they try to correct the perceived equilibrium disturbance by straightening themselves. In the process, they lose all control over their balance and fall to the ground. They do not become unconscious or nauseous, and they do remember the fall. After being stunned and temporarily immobilized, they are able to get up. Such an episode is called "otolithic crisis of Tumarkin," which is related to sudden mechanical malfunctions in the gravity sensors of the otoliths organs that house the ear rocks.

The second kind of drop attack described by Ménière's patients involves surprise vertigo or spinning episodes that are so sudden, so strong, and so immobilizing that those affected fall to the ground, totally helpless. Drop attacks — no matter what the cause — are scary events that undermine the people's self-confidence tremendously and endanger their safety most seriously. As there are other medical conditions that can lead to "sudden falls," it is important to report such episodes immediately to the physician for a proper evaluation.

Triggers, Aggravating Factors, and Auras

Discussions in group meetings always turn quite lively when it comes to sharing some of the triggers that set off or aggravate symptoms or possibly precipitate an attack. Flashing lights, waving hands, zany carpet or brick floor patterns, rapidly changing pictures such as TV ads or movie special effects all figure on the long list of things that often lead to an unpleasant experience. If I had to take a guess, I would say that serious vestibulooccular reflex (VOR) challenges can be the bane of many a Ménière's patient. While in the presence of people with Ménière's disease, it is important to speak slowly and calmly, as emoting with the hands or accentuating a statement with tons of body language could aggravate their symptoms, or worse, bring about an attack.

Another frequent topic for discussion is the possible effect that air pressure changes have on Ménière's disease. Many patients claim to be affected by weather-related barometric pressure variations, which can cause a worsening of symptoms if not a full-blown attack. Airplane rides test anyone's ears and eustachian tubes, but for those with Ménière's disease, air travel may be an attack waiting to happen. Although doctors tend to discount the barometric pressure theory, patients who are at the receiving end of ill effects disagree. I join their ranks. I know I have suffered some vestibular damage, and barometric pressure changes, especially sudden swings, seriously upset my well-being.

Ménière's attacks are exhausting events that test the resilience of those affected. After the symptoms ebb, people are extremely tired and just want to sleep. Wondering whether hearing will return to its pre-episode level seems to be a constant worry. Long-term effects include the possibility of gradual hearing loss as well as lingering equilibrium issues that might call for vestibular retraining therapy.

Some people can tell that an attack is coming on because they get an *aura*. Sensations that may herald an imminent episode include

148

hearing changes, feelings of increasing ear pressure, and low-frequency tinnitus noises such as a roaring or rumbling, as if an oncoming train or a tornado were bearing down on the ear. One lady described her ear prior to an attack as howling and being covered with plastic wrap, and her hearing as fading in and out.

So far, Ménière's disease is, by definition, idiopathic in nature. The underlying cause that leads to the collection of symptoms referred to as Ménière's disease is unknown. Although there are various theories, there is no clear-cut answer for the exact process of the condition.

Theories on Possible Causes

Ménière's disease is often referred to as "idiopathic endolymphatic hydrops." *Hydrops* is the excessive accumulation of fluid in body tissues or cavities. In this case, the fluid is the endolymph that fills the membranous labyrinth of the inner ear.

Ménière's disease is said to be the result of increasing and fluctuating endolymph levels in the inner ear. The fluid build-up swells the inner-ear hearing and balance ducts, which interferes with the ear's normal functions and can bring on symptoms and attacks. The true reason why the fluid levels rise is not known. It is thought, however, that various factors can lead to hydrops: an overproduction of endolymph; abnormalities in endolymph flow and absorption; and blockages of the drainage and pressure-equalizing structure made of the *endolymphatic duct and sac*. Surgical procedures aimed at decompressing this system can be performed in extreme cases.

Although the "increased endolymph pressure theory" is the commonly accepted explanation for this puzzling disorder, there is mounting controversy and debate among specialists regarding the origin of Ménière's disease. Scientists increasingly think that a variety of factors might contribute to the development of Ménière's symptoms. There are those who suspect a viral connection, while others wonder about an immune element involving the endolymphatic sac, a theory that is gaining in popularity. Suggestions that changes in the chemical composition of the endolymph might be to blame have raised interest. It has also been found that Ménière's disease can run in families. Genetic factors could account for immune response issues or abnormalities in the anatomy of the endolymph channel system. There is also great interest in investigating a possible link between Ménière's disease and migraines, as many Ménière's patients report a migraine history.

Dr. Ménière might be amazed to learn that the disorder that was named for him still baffles the medical and scientific communities so many years after he first described it.

Diagnosis

Because the symptoms associated with Ménière's disease could point to many other conditions, it is important to get a thorough medical checkup, preferably by a specialist. A detailed description of the symptoms, along with the patient's health, hearing, and family histories will guide the physician in the diagnostic efforts. The diagnostic menu for Ménière's disease is essentially the same as for SSHL. It features a full set of hearing assessments, a variety of blood tests, an MRI or CT scan of the head, and an involuntary rapid-eye movement (nystagmus) study known as an electronystagmography (ENG) or videonystagmography (VNG) test. In the end, the diagnosis comes down to *excluding* other causes for the symptoms, as there are no tests that are specific for Ménière's disease.

The ENG or VNG screens for problems in the pathways that connect the inner ears, the eyes, and the brain. The test consists of four distinct parts and checks for evidence of vestibular system and/ or neurological issues. The older ENG test uses electrodes that are attached to the skin around the eyes for the purpose of studying nystagmus. ENG has been largely replaced by a new version, the VNG. VNG is more precise and more comfortable for the patient than the ENG. It uses infrared cameras built into goggles for observing and measuring nystagmus directly—no more electrodes. The patient wears what looks like sci-fi headgear that allows the specialist to watch for specific eye movements. The nature and site of possible problems is often betrayed by the way the eyes jump, quiver, twitch, jerk, or roll. Although these tests are also not specific for Ménière's disease, they can give the doctor valuable clues on how to proceed and where to search next.

Managing the Symptoms of Ménière's Disease

The fact that Ménière's disease is such a multifaceted and unpredictable condition makes it tough to manage. It is difficult for the doctor to evaluate the success of a prescribed treatment regime because the severity of the symptoms does not follow a set pattern.

Efforts to control Ménière's disease are mostly aimed at inner-ear fluid pressure control. Patients are instructed on the "hydrops diet." This is basically a serious salt-restricted diet that also limits substances that can make symptoms worse. Caffeine, chocolate, nicotine, and sugar, as well as aspartame and MSG should be avoided. As food and environmental allergens have raised concerns, people are also encouraged to determine if other ingredients—dyes, wheat, dairy, gluten or even cleaning chemicals—might worsen their condition.

Extra rest and sleep are highly recommended and many patients express the need for "quiet time" on a regular basis. Meditation, relaxation techniques, carefully designed exercise programs, and adapted tai chi and yoga routines are said to have positive effects. Patients often report that balance training therapy is of great help. Eventually, people learn what to avoid and what *lifestyle changes* help manage the severity of the symptoms. Supporting the patient emotionally is also a major component of Ménière's disease care.

The major purpose for drug treatment is a multi-pronged effort to prevent dizziness, vertigo, and nausea and to ward off attacks.

Medications that are routinely called upon to help Ménière's disease patients belong to various categories. Diuretics are meant to lower overall fluid levels in an effort to control inner-ear endolymph levels. Vestibular sedatives prevent dizziness and vertigo, which also decreases the incidence of nausea. Anti-nauseants are standard fare for Ménière's disease patients for obvious reasons. Valium-related anti-anxiety drugs help calm the patient and decrease the incidence of vertigo by soothing an overactive vestibular apparatus. Medications from the corticosteroid family may be used, especially during attacks, as they suppress the immune system and decrease inner ear inflammation.

Guided by accepted treatment standards and medication side-effect profiles, specialists choose those medicines that are most helpful and appropriate for the individual. For patients, it is most important to understand *when* and *how* the different drugs are to be used: between attacks, during attacks, on a regular basis, or on an "as needed" basis.

In the end, what works best is determined by the patient's response to a personalized combination package of diet, medications, exercise, relaxation, and rest. Empathetic doctors and audiologists, as well as support groups, are also considered beneficial by many.

A prescription device is available meant to ease obstinate vertigo related to Ménière's. The strategy is to relieve inner-ear fluid pressure by delivering low-pressure air pulses to the ear. To make this possible, however, ventilation tubes must be installed in the eardrum, which is considered a surgical procedure. The air that is applied to the ear then travels through the tubes to the middle ear and on to the inner ear via the round window. In theory, the air puffs induce endolymph fluid movement, which in turn helps to equalize endolymph pressure. It is hard to predict whether this technique will bring relief. Yet the high price of the device and the need to insert tubes call for a serious conversation with the physician on the pros and cons of this type of treatment.

More serious interventions, including *surgery*, are reserved for those with severely debilitating vertigo that cannot be managed by other means. It is important for the patient to fully understand the proposed procedure and its possible benefits, side effects, and limitations. It is even more important to be under the care of a specialized physician with the most up-to-date knowledge of Ménière's disease, one who is familiar with the latest procedure protocols and with the newest techniques and who has plenty of experience in performing them. The approach that is taken depends a lot on whether the patient still has hearing in the affected ear, as well as the severity of the case.

Corticosteroids can be instilled or injected into the ear in an attempt to curb severe symptoms. As mentioned, they decrease inflammation and are helpful if an immune component is suspected. In order to stop disabling dizziness, the doctor can take advantage of the ototoxic effects of the antibiotic gentamicin by skillfully injecting the drug into the affected ear. This procedure is called a "chemical labyrinthectomy." As gentamicin is more toxic to the vestibular system than to the hearing organ, it is hoped that a targeted "poisoning" of the vestibular system will prevent dizziness, while preserving whatever hearing is left in the ear. Alternatively, if only one ear is affected, if the patient has lost all hearing in that ear, and if all other attempts at relief have failed, the whole inner ear can be surgically removed in an effort to alleviate symptoms. This intervention, which does not preserve hearing in any way, is known as a "surgical labyrinthectomy."

For easing pressure, surgical decompression procedures aimed at the endolymphatic sac can also be considered. During an "endolymphatic sac enhancement," the surgeon carves out some of the surrounding bone, which provides more room for the sac to expand in response to endolymph pressure surges. Sac enhancement eases pressure on the structure without causing injury.

A decompression that involves puncturing the sac for the purpose of draining off fluid is also done. This can be a one-time intervention, or it can be accompanied by the placement of a drainage "shunt," or tube, for further reducing pressure by diverting excess endolymph away from the ear.

In people with normal or near-normal hearing who have failed to respond to any attempts at symptom relief, a delicate procedure is to cut or sever the vestibular or balance portion of the eighth cranial nerve while leaving the hearing portion intact. This is called a "vestibular nerve section." Obviously, any of these interventions are reserved for advanced, extreme cases and warrant an in-depth discussion with the specialist.

PART THREE
WHEN HEARING LOSS IS ONLY THE BEGINNING

Chapter 24
Tinnitus

The day after my ear incident I was admitted to the hospital for tests, nausea control, and blood electrolyte corrections. At some time during the night, I began to "hear" an occasional strange noise in my deaf left ear. This was definitively not normal. At first it sounded like a very low-frequency, slurred murmur that reminded me of a B-grade movie villain's voice. The following morning, however, it was a much more pronounced whir that was difficult to ignore. I would soon find out that there was a lot more to hearing loss than not hearing so well; hearing loss can be accompanied by a variety of other features.

As I stated earlier, when Dr. Todd came to visit me in the hospital, I reported "hearing" all sorts of odd sounds. He told me that, regrettably, I was developing subjective tinnitus as a consequence of my hearing loss. He had so hoped that I would be spared. He used the term "subjective" because I alone could "hear" the sounds. He informed me that these were "phantom" noises that came from the brain, not the ear. Some people perceive the sounds in the ears, while others perceive that they come more from inside the head and refer to them as "head noise." Although tinnitus is frequently a *symptom* of other underlying conditions, in my case we knew what caused it—cochlear and possibly nerve damage.

Dr. Todd mentioned that many people with hearing loss report having tinnitus. This is when I learned that the appearance of ear noises is often the first sign—*a red flag*—that something is not right with our hearing. The doctor felt that my noises would change, as the sounds of tinnitus tend to match the frequencies of the hearing loss.

Over the next few days, the garbled noises gave indeed way to more generic din that gradually became refined to a high-frequency hiss.

The doctor was cautiously optimistic that the noises might ease a bit as I regained more hearing, but I should not count on it. He said that unfortunately there was no cure for tinnitus but that various management approaches could make life easier. This was bad news. I could not imagine how I would ever live with tinnitus, my "ear phantom," after it besieged my damaged ear within hours of my hearing loss.

Tinnitus is defined as the perception of sound in the absence of an outside noise source. It is commonly called "ringing in the ears." The name itself is derived from the Latin verb *tinnire*, which means "to ring." This is, however, a very limited description. It did not take long for me to learn that there was a lot more to tinnitus than mere ringing.

It was depressing to hear Dr. Todd say that there was no cure for the ear din. Many different causes are known to trigger this mysterious condition, yet it is unclear exactly how the noises are generated, why they are generated, and by what nervous pathways they travel. Until we know that, it will be difficult to devise a medication or some other treatment able to quiet the phantom. Scientists agree that the answers are within the brain, which is a simple but very loaded truth. We need more research and for that we need money, a lot of devoted scientists, and loads of sophisticated equipment. Although it is being studied worldwide, the phantom does not surrender its secrets easily.

Tracking the Tinnitus Signal

There are plenty of theories about the nature of tinnitus but none gives any definitive answers. Considering the variety of causes that can lead to tinnitus, it is unlikely that a single theory could explain it all. The suspected mechanisms are not mutually exclusive, and more than one of them might contribute to the ear noise in any given case.

A amaged cochlea has long been considered a leading cause of tinnitus. If hearing cells are harmed, they send frequency impulses to the brain that are faulty, random, and weak. An injured cochlear nerve might similarly relay defective frequency information or stop transmitting signals altogether. In the process, the nicely organized frequency map of the auditory cortex is seriously disrupted. The attempt of the brain to tune into the frequencies that have weakened or fallen off the grid may ultimately result in tinnitus noise that matches the affected frequencies, which is certainly true in my case. Though cochlear damage might get the tinnitus ball rolling, it has been shown that once the noises take hold, they seem to feed on themselves. There are areas in the brain that actually change in response to long term tinnitus.

Scientists realized early on that cochlear issues were only part of the tinnitus puzzle. The search had to be expanded beyond the inner ear to include the intricacies of the auditory pathways, the brainstem, and the auditory cortex, or hearing portion of the brain.

Researchers have identified a sound-relay structure in the brain— the dorsal cochlear nucleus (DCN)—as a target for study. Over the years, suspicions have mounted that changes in DCN nervous activity contribute to the generation of tinnitus signals. It also has been found that the DCN has ties to other areas of the brain, notably to those that are in involved with concentration and emotions. This is significant. Anyone who has tinnitus knows that especially negative emotions and paying too much attention to the noise can whip the phantom into action. It sounds reasonable that the DCN will be a focal point when scientists look for ways of treating tinnitus effectively. At this time, research centering on the DCN and its role in tinnitus is ongoing and very lively.

By using a variety of high-tech diagnostic machines, researchers also peek into the revved-up tinnitus brain to measure and record responses. Functional MRI scans (f MRI) have revealed important information on how tinnitus signals travel and which brain structures might play a part in the generation and maintenance of the tinnitus sounds.

In addition, scientists are working their way from identifiable anatomical details to the cellular levels. Special proteins, calcium channels, receptors, and brain substances are all put under the microscope in order to determine their contribution to the ear ruckus. Some scientists believe that the paths traveled by tinnitus signals, no matter what their cause, intersect at a common point. Locating such a convergence point could be of great importance when it comes to developing drugs capable of stopping the noises in their tracks.

Those who are interested in the more intricate scientific research details may find *Tinnitus Today,* a publication of the American Tinnitus Association (ATA), most interesting. Thanks to unrelenting research efforts, we know a lot more today than we did just a few years ago. New diagnostic technology has been of great assistance. Also, the ever-increasing number of tinnitus patients seeking help tells researchers that this is indeed a field that deserves their attention; millions of us are waiting. Maybe at some point in our lives, we will enjoy once again a bit of quiet, thanks to all of those who so tirelessly stalk the phantom on our behalf.

Chapter 25
Tinnitus Types and the Importance
of a Medical Evaluation

Various types of tinnitus produce a variety of different noises. Our being able to describe our ear sounds accurately might lead the physician in the right direction when looking for a possible cause.

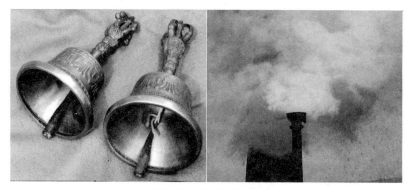

Although tinnitus is often called "ringing in the ears," many describe different sounds. People with tinnitus often say that they hear ringing, buzzing, steam hissing or other sounds. *photos: R.Hammond*

Subjective Tinnitus

When Dr. Todd initiated me to the reality that the ear phantom had come to live with me, he called the noises "subjective tinnitus." This is the most widespread type of tinnitus. One could call it the classic kind. Most cases are due to "sensorineural" hearing loss, which is often the result of damage due to excess noise. The American Tinnitus Association states that more than 90 percent of their members with tinnitus report some degree of hearing loss.

"Subjective" means that the noises can only be "heard" by the patient. Even with special instruments, the doctor cannot verify the sounds. They are whatever the patient reports them to be, which makes them subjective in nature. I wondered what types of situations might set us up for subjective tinnitus and found that the list of possibilities is a long one.

Anything that damages the cochlea, the cochlear nerve, and other auditory nervous pathways will lead to hearing loss and possibly tinnitus. The insults might be due to excess noise, viral infections, ototoxic substances, ear or head injuries, tumors, autoimmune disorders, Ménière's disease, or even the aging process. Anything that physically interferes with or blocks sound transmission to the brain can trigger tinnitus. Ear wax plugs, middle ear fluid accumulation due to infection, middle ear growths, and problems involving the ossicle chain, such as otosclerosis, all can generate tinnitus. In some cases the noises may be linked to vitamin deficiencies, such as vitamin B-12. Anxiety and depression can even unleash the phantom. There are, however, instances when tinnitus is idiopathic because the reason for the noises cannot be determined, even after thorough medical investigations.

As the causes for subjective tinnitus run the gamut from ear wax to tumors, it is important never to ignore the noise. Quite a few subjective tinnitus triggers are treatable. Therefore, any abnormal ear or head sounds are best evaluated by a specialist, such as an ENT doctor or otologist.

What does subjective tinnitus *sound* like? Michelangelo was plagued by the constant chirping of crickets. The composer Ludwig van Beethoven wrote that his ears whistled and buzzed continually. Everybody seems to "hear" something different—ringing, buzzing, whistling, hissing, humming, roaring, howling, etc. Any and all sounds are possible. If the noise barrage is even, it becomes easier to ignore it after a while, at least in theory.

I have high-frequency hearing loss. My tinnitus sounds like a wall of high-pitched hissing splattered with on-and-off outbursts of even higher frequencies or crackling noises. Now and then I am treated to the jolly popping of bubble wrap. Siren-type howls really scared me for a while. I felt like I was in a Parisian ambulance. Oooah-oooah! The sounds would appear suddenly, for no good reason, and like any sounds of a pulsing nature, they were very hard to ignore. This has not happened for a while, however, and I am grateful for that. I have learned not to freak out too fast when additional superimposed noises pop up. Thankfully, they tend to fade away, and then I am back to my familiar wall of hissing.

Some people may perceive other ear noises that are more complicated than the simple hissing or buzzing sounds of regular tinnitus. These are often elderly people with longstanding hearing loss and frequently also subjective tinnitus. In the absence of obvious external sources, they report hearing heavy equipment at work, such as snowplows in July, or noises that have a talking, singing, or musical quality to them. "Voices" might be recognizable, but they are distorted and the chatter is without meaningful content. Also, the voices do *not* "talk" to the people or about them, as in certain psychiatric conditions. The musical and singing tunes can be fuzzy or sometimes quite clear, to the point where it is possible to "Name That Tune." There are those who perceive such puzzling sounds on a regular basis, while others become aware of them occasionally. People are not eager to discuss these noises because they are afraid of being considered mentally affected. These *complex phantom noises* are not considered in the regular tinnitus category. Instead, they are referred to as *auditory hallucinations*.

A hallucination is anything that the brain perceives in the absence of a physical source. Ultimately, the many sounds of subjective tinnitus are also hallucinations, with the exception that those sounds are *simple* in nature. There is nobody hissing into my ear, but I "hear" it, 24/7. Yet the term "hallucination" carries an unwelcome stigma. Hearing loss specialist Neil Bauman, PhD, offers a different terminology: he refers to these ear hallucinations as "musical ear syndrome."

People with auditory hallucinations must check on the possible cause with an ear specialist. Just like regular tinnitus, this could be due to many things. It could be a consequence of hearing loss. It could be due to a lack of sound stimulation, and living in a less quiet environment might help. It is important, however, to be sure that it is not related to a more serious cause, such as a brain lesion or tumor.

Loud bangs that seem to come from the outside environment but are actually generated inside the head often go unreported as tinnitus. These are isolated, very loud, explosion-type sounds that sometimes blast away just as an individual dozes off or wakes up. I had two of these within the first few years of my ear event. Once, I jumped out of bed, sure that a shot had been fired at very close range. My husband was awake and reading. I asked if he had heard "that shot." He gave me a strange look and stated that he had not heard a thing. For a moment, I wondered which one of us had a hearing loss, yet I became suspicious of my ears. What was wrong now? When I went for another hearing test, I asked the audiologist, but she did not have an explanation. The audiogram did not show any changes, which was good. Regardless, I kept searching until I finally found a reference that mentioned these rather unsettling events. Balance and hearing expert, neurologist Timothy C. Hain, MD, tells about the "exploding head syndrome." The salvos are supposedly due to non-dangerous, brief seizures in the auditory cortex—the hearing sector of the brain.

Asking people to describe the *loudness* of their tinnitus will draw very subjective responses. Tinnitus noise levels can vary from mild to aggressive, which makes for better days and not-so-good days. On rare occasions at the start, my buzz could be so soft that I had hope that it might go away. Then, for whatever reason, it would surge and become quite loud and obnoxious again. Eventually, it found its pace, and now it is mostly tolerable. However, there are those days when it is a real challenge not to let the ear phantom spoil my good humor.

Overall, for most people the annoyance meter fluctuates between tolerable and being driven to distraction. For tinnitus patients, it is important to determine what revs up the noise and what settles it down. Often, it is not so much the loudness that bothers me; it's the *unrelenting* hissing that gets to me.

Somatic or "Body" Tinnitus

In Greek, the word "soma" refers to the body. Researchers have suspected for some time that in certain people, subjective tinnitus has a somatic, or body, component to it. Indeed, there are nerve connections between the hearing centers and body pressure and body movement sensors located in skin, muscles, and joints. The way these two systems interact in the brain forms the basis for the tinnitus/ somatic connection. The discovery of the existence of such a somatic element has opened up a whole new area for studying the nature and origin of tinnitus and for focusing on its nerve networks. Once more, researchers suspect that the DCN (dorsal cochlear nucleus) plays a mediator role in this phenomenon.

Due to body sensor activation, people who have *certain physical conditions* can have severe tinnitus in the absence of hearing loss. Issues related to areas of the head, neck, back, and jaw, such as head and neck injuries, dental problems, whiplash, cervical disc issues, or temporomandibular joint (TMJ) dysfunction fall into this category. It is important to note that these conditions are associated with at least a fair amount of muscle tension and strain. TMJ patients can relate many of their symptoms to teeth clenching and jaw pressure. Ideally, the noises should go away or ease once the underlying problem is successfully treated, but that is often a lot easier said than done.

Some years ago it was found that in certain patients with existing tinnitus, it was possible to change the way they perceived the loudness or pitch of the noises by stimulating a nerve in the arm. Although it seems mighty weird, it was this crucial observation that led scientists to suspect a link between tinnitus and body sensors. Once they began investigating, they found that roughly two-thirds of tinnitus patients could *change the pitch and/or loudness* of their noises by performing certain movements or body manipulations, such as clenching their teeth, opening their jaw, contracting certain muscles, moving their eyes, or by applying pressure to areas of the head or neck region. When talking to people who have the ability to soothe their tinnitus by somatic means, it becomes clear that everybody has a different special "trick."

For example, a friend of mine with a low-frequency hearing loss, who has had tinnitus for years, is able to lower the perceived loudness by applying pressure with her fingertip to the outer portion of her ear canal. Generally, the tinnitus does not bother her outrageously, but on bad days such a technique comes in handy. This won't work for everyone, and it does not work for me.

Somatic links, however, can also seriously sour the ear phantom's mood and work to the disadvantage of patients. I met a gentleman who was unable to move his eyes upward without sending his tinnitus into orbit. He gave up driving because any craning of the neck had a similar effect.

The issue of the somatic/tinnitus connections presents researchers with some challenging questions but also with some interesting learning opportunities. By studying people capable of altering their noises, they hope to gain insights into the inner workings of the tinnitus process, as well as some understanding of how the signal is generated in the brain.

Objective Tinnitus

Unlike subjective tinnitus, objective tinnitus *can* be heard or in some way be detected by a specialist with the right equipment. One type of tinnitus that is objective in nature is "pulsatile" tinnitus, so called because there is usually a rhythmic quality to these noises, like a heartbeat. Expressions used to describe the sounds include whooshing, swishing, pulsing, pounding, humming, rushing, or thumping. These sounds are often related to blood circulation issues, such as high blood pressure, misshapen blood vessels, blood flow turbulence, reduced blood viscosity or stickiness, a blood vessel that presses on a nerve connected with hearing, hardening of the arteries, or even aneurysms.

Major blood vessels lie close enough to the ears that blood movement within these vessels can become audible. For example, the patient might be able to hear the rushing and pulsing as blood is being forced through narrowed vessels, sounds that can also be detected by the practitioner. People who hear the gushing of their blood or the pumping of their hearts should find out *at once* what the problem might be. Their ears are giving them hints that should not be ignored. Although there are those cases that remain mysteries even after lengthy investigations, we should not give up.

The December 2007 issue of the magazine *Tinnitus Today* published a telling letter from a reader who had been diagnosed with pulsatile tinnitus—"the form a person hears with every heartbeat"— some two and a half years back. She was consistently told that there was no cure, but she persisted. She ended up doing her own research and found an article that recommended that people with tinnitus might consider seeing a neurologist. She did just that. The neurologist ordered a CT scan that finally shed some light on the issue. Her problem was a leaky arteriovenous malformation (AVM), an abnormal tangle of veins and arteries. The noise in her ear was blood leaking from one of the vessels. Surgery plugged the drip, and she reported that afterward she felt fine and was noise-free.

A man told me that he was driven to distraction by listening to unrelenting blood pumping action in one ear. He went to an ENT, who referred him to a cardiovascular specialist. After a variety of tests, he had a "Roto-Rooter" procedure done—I imagine he had plaque cleaned out of his blood vessels—and the problem resolved itself gradually. He was put on a diet and exercise regime and given cholesterol pills. Today, he looks great.

Other objective tinnitus noises include those related to issues with the eustachian tube and to *spasms* of muscles of the soft palate and of the middle ear. Eustachian tubes that are stuck in the "open" position can contribute to ocean-roar sounds in the ears that vary with breathing. Rapid, rhythmic, clicking sounds can be brought on by contractions of the soft palate muscles in the back of the mouth. Twitches of the stapedius muscle are said to produce high-pitched tics that can be audible by means of specialized equipment. Yet stapedius spasms have also been described as causing crackling or rumbling noises. Frenzied contractions of the tensor tympani generate thumping-type sounds that cause the eardrum to pulsate and can be seen and heard by the specialist. This interesting fact rang a bell with me. Might an overactive tensor tympani have been the reason for those intermittent, rapid-fire, dull popping noises that I heard in my left ear during our Alaska cruise? Although I mentioned the rather unsettling symptom to my doctors during my first visit with them, I never found out for sure if the noises were relevant to my case or what might have set them off.

Typewriter or Staccato Tinnitus

This type of tinnitus is characterized by sounds reminiscent of popcorn bursts, typewriter tapping, machine-gun sounds, or Morse code. The noises are intermittent and often quite loud. They come on abruptly and affect one ear. In some cases the bursts have been triggered by certain head positions or by loud noise. Researchers believe that typewriter tinnitus may be related to irritability or hyperactivity of the eighth cranial nerve. This type of tinnitus has responded to the medication carbamazepine (Tegretol).

***

Need for a Medical Check: Ignorance is not Bliss

We should never simply just ignore tinnitus. As a potential symptom of an underlying condition, any ear noise is best investigated by an ear specialist. Besides hearing loss and the conditions that cause it, there are numerous other possible tinnitus triggers, some of which can be treated or fixed. We owe it to ourselves to find out if the phantom sounds spell bad news, or if they are merely an annoyance. Even if no definite cause is found, knowing what does *not* cause them can be tremendously reassuring.

Any consultation with a physician is a dialogue for which we must prepare. As patients we are called upon to be reliable historians, but we must not forget to also be effective interviewers. Asking questions of our health care professionals is part of the process. When initiating a tinnitus workup, the doctor usually checks on the more obvious causes first. A physical, an ear inspection, and a complete set of audiometric or hearing tests are a good start.

For our part, it is important to give *an accurate description of the sounds* and to plot a detailed sequence of events—when and how the noises first began, or if they can be linked to any special circumstances, such as loud noise exposures, a recent illness, stress, anxiety, depression, or a new medicine or supplement. We should also take all medications and health care products to the appointment for the doctor to review.

The Art of Perseverance

When calling an ENT specialist group for an appointment, it is good to ask for their tinnitus, ear, and hearing *expert*—we want and need the best. Within the same clinic, doctors usually have their own field of specialization. This is why it is important to find *the* physician who has a particular interest in tinnitus, who understands the ear phantom, who keeps up with the latest information, and who looks into the case no matter how the condition can or cannot be treated.

Tracking tinnitus is like finding one's way in a maze. It is often lengthy, frustrating work for both the doctor and the patient, but we do not want to miss anything.

That said, the statement that "nothing can be done" keeps hanging on in the medical community. Consequently, many people who try to find answers come away from their medical appointments somewhat defeated and wondering if theirs is a lost cause. Health insurance restrictions have been cited for patients' lack of physician choice. In the hopefully unlikely event that a doctor shows little interest in our case, we might ask for a *referral* to an ear/tinnitus specialist for an evaluation and consult. We must not surrender. Remember the story about the woman with the pulsatile tinnitus who did not accept that "nothing could be done"? She did her own research, and what she learned probably saved her life. There are times when it pays to persevere.

Chapter 26
Tinnitus Management Basics

When I got home from the hospital, reality began to sink in. My doctors held out hope that my hearing might eventually improve somewhat, yet there were no guarantees. Everything that could be done had been done. As hearing loss was the cause of my tinnitus, the thought that the phantom had taken up permanent residence in my ear struck a note of desperation in me. I knew that there was no "cure" in the form of a pill or other type of treatment, but Dr. Todd had mentioned that certain "management techniques" could ease the ear cacophony. At the time, I was overwhelmed by the events and had no clue what was meant by "management techniques." Gradually, I came to the realization that I needed to get a lot more information. The attempt to put some chinks in the phantom's armor put me on yet another fascinating leg of an already amazing journey.

Reactions and Attitudes

After medical checks fail to identify an underlying treatable or fixable cause, all tinnitus sufferers face the challenge of *dealing* with the noises in order to maintain their quality of life. Dealing with tinnitus goes beyond coping with it. To me, "coping" suggests an almost passive surrender to the ear phantom, whereas "dealing" implies taking an active role to gain an edge over him. The goal for dealing with tinnitus is to increase the number of good or better days by becoming as phantom-neutral in our responses as possible. This is quite a task, as every tinnitus case is different, yet specialists point out that our attitude and reaction to the noise can make all the difference in the world.

Some people just have tinnitus. It is like any other noise and does not elicit an overly emotional response. Then there are those, like me, for whom it makes life at times quite miserable and who tend to harbor negative emotions toward it. This type of attitude, however, can seriously empower the phantom—I found that out the hard way. Obsessing over my tinnitus and fighting what could not be changed did not help me gain control so that I could move forward. The more I resisted, the louder the din became. As I learned more, I began to understand that the aim was to curb my balky responses and to develop strategies that would let me accept my ear noises and live with them without surrendering to them.

A few million tinnitus patients in the United States are debilitated by the condition. Not only does tinnitus ruin their quality of life, but it runs their life. These are often people whose noises are very loud or of a nature that makes them difficult to ignore. I got a taste of such a situation when I had episodes of cadenced French siren-type sounds. Another noise that sometimes tests my resilience is an extremely high, bone-sawing frequency that fortunately fades—at least it has so far.

Of course, everybody must make their own decisions. I believe, however, that people who are beset by an unruly, overbearing phantom to the point that they have trouble carrying on a daily routine need to consult at once with a tinnitus expert. Quick professional interventions can stem the torture. In the short-term, medication might help tame the overwhelming anxiety that so often consumes the patient. The important thing is to seek help immediately. Before we can begin to deal with our ear noises, we must gain control over ourselves.

A Most Revealing Lecture

When I first heard the sounds of my unrelenting, buzzing tinnitus, life stopped in its tracks. I was devastated. I suddenly had visions of heading into a box canyon with no way out and no way back. There was no place to hide from the hissing that pursued me relentlessly, day and night. It took a toll on my quality of life. My productivity nose-dived. How was I ever going to live with this? How could I bring at least some normalcy back into my life?

One day, a doctor spoke to my tinnitus support group, and his statements made a great deal of sense. He came at a good time for me. I was done with the fighting and the groaning; I was willing to listen and learn.

First, he stressed the importance and advantages of having the noises checked out medically. Treating or fixing any contributing aggravations might already bring great relief. Then, he wove tinnitus management principles, many of which were already familiar to me, into a recipe that I could understand. He talked about two major components in the process of gaining control over the phantom: de-conditioning and habituation. We can learn, he said, to "park the noise" and to turn tinnitus into a non-issue. We were cautioned, however, that these slow, gradual processes would happen deep inside of us, on a subconscious level, and were not simply mind-over-matter efforts.

De-conditioning is the first step if we want to soothe our attitude toward tinnitus. A change in attitude will not happen, however, if our negative perceptions of tinnitus loudness and annoyance continue unchecked. De-conditioning involves the breaking of some bad habits. Our unyielding demeanor, fears, and misconceptions have programmed or conditioned the brain to react with hurtful emotions to the ear clamor. We let tinnitus dominate us and concentrate way too much on it. The more we dwell on it, the worse it gets. These practices do not help our cause, however, as they further increase our stress levels, and stress is known to worsen tinnitus. Identifying situations that turn up the volume on the sounds is very helpful during de-conditioning. Learning how to manage stress, relax, avoid silence, and focus our minds away from the ear din help curb our tinnitus obsession and reflex anti-tinnitus reactions. During de-conditioning, we essentially give the brain a chance to purge itself of counterproductive responses so that it can desensitize to the sounds and eventually habituate to them. Although the noise remains, our attitude toward it and our perception of it will slowly change. The ideal plan is for the brain to shift into a reaction-neutral mode whenever we are confronted with tinnitus annoyance.

Habituation basically means that we adapt to the sounds, as the level of arousal that the ear phantom can unleash decreases. The noises will still be there, but they will have lost their meaning. They will bother us a lot less, maybe even not at all.

Education also can help us de-condition. Any knowledge of tinnitus basics often greatly lessens anxiety and misguided beliefs. Certainly, there is still much to be studied and researched, but a lot is already known about some practical aspects of tinnitus, such as triggers and aggravating factors.

We were encouraged to ask experts for answers and explanations to which we can relate. After all, the purpose in educating patients is to help them better understand the nature of their problem; in this case, tinnitus. Once that happens, it becomes much easier to deal with the ear noise realities. Learning the facts gradually loosens the grip that the phantom has on us. For me, it unhitched a major portion of the emotional burden that I had come to attach to the noises. As my perception changed, the tinnitus conundrum shifted onto a more neutral, scientific ground.

There are many other benefits to becoming informed. Getting a grasp of the hearing and tinnitus fundamentals turns us into better communicators with our health care specialists. It teaches us to formulate relevant questions regarding our condition, possible treatments, and future outlook. Learning also makes us curious as we begin to study the performance of our own phantom, what makes it soar, and what soothes it. This is significant. If we can identify and manage triggers, we could well have more peaceful days. Any success encourages us to stay on the path that will eventually lead us toward habituation.

As the doctor spoke, I realized that my coming to grips with the phantom would take commitment, time, and discipline and would be a lengthy process—it was and still is. Although the structured approach sounded logical, I stood in front of a mountainous assignment. Would it be feasible to tackle this on my own? Yet for the first time, I saw a chance to extricate myself from the clutches of the tinnitus ghost sounds. But first, I had to figure out how this new information applied to my life and how it would influence my efforts for taming my ear phantom.

The doctor was right; over time I had taught my brain plenty of contrary responses toward tinnitus. I continued to associate it with the terrible day when my left ear got whacked and my life changed forever. Deep down, the part of the brain in charge of emotions had become conditioned to react with depression, frustration, anger, and resentment to the ever-present sounds. If I was to win a round or two in this battle, I had to kick my chaotic feelings down a few notches. Then, by taming myself I would eventually tame the phantom. Even though it might take a while before I would reap the fruits of my labor, the important thing would be to stick with the plan and not give up.

Accepting What I Could Not Change

Before I could proceed with any actions, I had to get out of my resentment mode, let go of obstructionist sentiments and reactions, and look at the reality of my situation. Once I had taken stock, I realized that I had put myself through a lot of anguish over circumstances that were totally out of my control. The bottom line was that my hearing would not improve much more and that the tinnitus would never go away. As a matter of fact, it might become worse with age and further hearing loss, yet I could not change that I was aging. Although barometric pressure swings affected both my tinnitus and balance, I could not change weather patterns either. These were the simple yet hard truths that I had to accept—without fuss. After the doctor's speech, I made a promise to myself to move on and not to live my life bemoaning what should be or what might have been, what was fair and what was not.

Ultimately, acceptance turned out to be a liberating experience that showed me that I was not totally powerless after all. I would use the energy that I wasted on being obstinate for learning as much as possible about my ear noises and for crafting preventive strategies that would make living together easier.

Trigger Management and Lifestyle Changes

I determined early on that stress, fatigue, loud noise, barometric pressure variations, and anxiety would drive the phantom into orbit. It was reassuring to find out that these triggers are commonly cited by tinnitus patients. In order to garner more peaceful days, I had to find ways to work around risk situations that could worsen the tinnitus din. This was especially important in the beginning. I needed to score some success that would encourage me to continue on the road to habituation. I compiled a list of aggravating factors and found that I actually had quite a bit of sway over some of them. I came to that recognition, once I understood that tinnitus has ties to the emotional systems of the brain. Although I might not have control over every situation in my life, I did have control over myself, my reactions, and my attitudes. If I could manage those, I might be able to dampen the annoyance. It was worth a try. I am actually amazed how much of a difference lifestyle and attitude tweaks have made.

Improving My Diet

Smarter dietary choices actually counted among my long-term health goals and became a roundabout way to check the tinnitus long term. Because cochlear damage is often due to ravages by free radicals, I have increased my intake of antioxidants. I eat a greater variety of vegetables, fruits, and berries, and I do so consistently. I also take a daily vitamin and antioxidant supplement. It is difficult to tell if these actions work, because the benefits are not immediately measurable. Yet it makes sense to me. In theory, anything that protects my hearing also prevents the tinnitus from worsening. So far, my audiogram has remained stable, and I feel better physically.

I greatly reduced my consumption of anything that reportedly kicks the brain into gear, such as excess sugar or chocolate, regular coffee, and tea, as well as the artificial sweetener aspartame. The body metabolizes aspartame into aspartate, a substance that acts as a brain stimulant. I also harbor a healthy fear of monosodium glutamate (MSG), another brain activator as well as a generous salt source. This flavor-enhancer, however, seems to be everywhere, and I do my very best to avoid it.

Besides its adverse cardiovascular effects, nicotine is also known to trigger or aggravate tinnitus.

Minding Medications

I took a good look at all my medications, both prescribed and over-the-counter but did not identify any particular offenders. Yet I notified my pharmacy to mark my records so that they would help me monitor any prescriptions for ototoxicity. As I mentioned earlier, such effects are often not listed in the patient pamphlets and need a more in-depth search of the professional databases. As medications can be changed and dosages can be adjusted, it is very important to let the prescriber know if we suspect a drug produces tinnitus or makes it worse.

Managing Noise

Loud noise always was a phenomenal stress-inducer for me. As already stated, an excessively loud noise exposure is also to blame for a good portion of my hearing loss. Now, there was an added fea-

177

ture—it aggravated my ear phantom. I could not retire from society, however, simply because there were situations that caused me ear-din distress. I soon realized that unless I wanted to turn into a hermit, I had to come up with a workable approach.

Short term, I had to minimize my tinnitus, while long term, I had to protect my hearing from further loss and therefore from further tinnitus boosts. I first learned to become more aware of the noise level in restaurants. Noise-related issues that always had been part of my dining experiences now cut seriously into my social life. Most restaurants became off limits to me during rush hours, and they still are. As part of my new strategies, I meet friends and business contacts for a late breakfast or an early lunch when the places are less frantic. Usually, I arrive early and try to garner a table that is *not* located next to the kitchen or by the bar. I also aim to stay away from loudspeakers. In older establishments this is often possible, but newer or refurbished places are peppered with these noise polluters. I have been known to ask, gently and politely, for the music to be turned down. Sometimes, it even works. Most of all, I never forget my earplugs, and on airplanes I always use noise-reducing headphones.

Avoiding Total Silence

Although loud noise is not appreciated by tinnitus sufferers, total silence also is not beneficial. I soon realized that when everything was really still, the only thing I heard was the tinnitus. The ear noise became my only focus, which often made for a distressing increase in volume. Then I learned that it is strongly recommended that we *not* spend hours on end in total silence. The most common noise for distracting a tinnitus patient is the use of white noise, or broadband noise, which is a sound blend rich in high-end frequencies. Although white noise is quite helpful, I prefer soothing nature tunes to help me focus my attention away from the hissing.

Total silence becomes a real challenge at night. We do want

noise, yet this is not the time for rock songs or opera. There are those who tune to the white noise of an off-the-air radio station. They may find the continuous static noise more agreeable than the tinnitus itself, and it helps them to drift off eventually. Those who want to be more advanced might invest in a white-noise generator. Some models are small enough for travel. White-noise CDs, relaxation-music CDs, and speaker-equipped pillows that can be plugged into any noise source are also for sale and might make a thoughtful gift for a tinnitus sufferer dear to us. I have a high-speed fan blowing year-round. Although the steady whir does not cover up my phantom, it does take the edge off. Then again, fans drive other people crazy. We are all different.

Managing Tension and Stress

As noted earlier, many tinnitus patients, including me, report that stress, tension, fatigue, and anxiety make the ear din worse. Louder and more aggressive noises, however, lead to even greater patient anxiety, resentment, and even desperation. Unfortunately, such reactions feed the ear phantom even more, and we are caught in a loop. In order to get a grip on tinnitus, the challenge is to settle down the emotional responses and to calm the body and the mind.

Most of us have our own foolproof ways for reining in the nerves: meditation, yoga, tai chi, prayer, water therapy, reading, music, walking, exercising, or biofeedback—whatever works. As I still have one ear that allows me to listen to music without distortions, I find slow, low-impact music—no lyrics, no orchestras—most helpful for my relaxation purposes. I love listening to nature sounds. The crashing of lake or ocean waves, the rushing of a brook, the call of the loon, the wind in the trees all take me on a virtual trip out of the mayhem and the stress, and whisk me to a different level of awareness. I fall asleep in the chair, which is totally unusual for me. Amazingly enough, before I had hearing loss and tinnitus, this type of music had little appeal for me. That said, because of their type and degree of hearing loss, many people do not get any benefit from music therapy. Instead, the sounds are too distant, tinny, and distorted to be helpful. They can become grating, which further aggravates a person's tension and ear ruckus.

Whenever the phantom becomes too obstreperous, I rely on my noise-reducing headphones to provide me with extra peace. Although they work for me, they do not help everyone, by far. When used by itself, noise-reduction wear actually dampens hearing and heightens the buzz, *but* if I enrich the sound environment by plugging in some soft tunes, it feels soothing to my brain. The outside noise is greatly reduced, while I hear the music a lot more clearly. I can listen at a lower volume than I would with a regular headset. Although the end result is a calming of my tinnitus, I also get the impression that I hear more evenly. The dulling, distorting, garbling effect due to my left hearing loss seems to be eased, which gives me the perception of hearing in stereo—at least somewhat. When wearing my noise-reducing headphones, I live in my own world and almost feel like my old self.

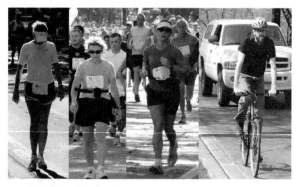

Exercising to one's ability reduces tension & stress for many. *photos: R.Hammond*

Exercising Regularly

Another way of taming tension and stress is to exercise regularly according to one's physical ability. I do not have any heart and joint issues, so my doctor gave me the green light to do whatever I like, within reason. I feel that my aerobic exercycle workout lifts my spirits as it gives me much needed energy and strength. Weather permitting, my husband and I also go for a daily walk in the neighborhood.

Managing Fatigue

Life with hearing loss, balance problems, and tinnitus can turn into an endurance test in no time at all. I tire easily and my reaction time slows down. As I become weary, the phantom becomes animated. Although my condition has improved somewhat, my best time of the day is still in the morning. Fatigue management forced me to rethink my daily schedule, and I reorganized my agenda accordingly. I schedule any meeting for the morning or early afternoon hours, if at all possible. I prioritize my work and do my house chores in stages. I balance activity with breaks, as best I can.

Since I sleep poorly, I added tinnitus distraction to my bedtime routine. I listen to relaxing sounds and read something calming. I also accepted that now and then it is okay to take a short daytime nap, which is a new experience for me and yet another truth that I had to accept.

Fighting Inactivity

An often forgotten antidote for tinnitus is to be active and to not focus on the ear din. Concentrating on other activities distracts us and so the tinnitus annoyance wanes. While wrestling with the phantom, many people forget about the rest of the world—their hobbies, their interests, their social contacts, their families. It happened to me. Tinnitus and the shock of the hearing loss robbed me of all initiative. I was so tired. I listened to the buzz all day long. I had not yet learned that the more I let myself be ruled by tinnitus, the more my life ground to a halt. Had my grandmother been here, she would have told me to "go and do something else."

Once I increased my activity level and was no longer totally engulfed by the ear noise, the fatigue eased and my mood and outlook on life improved. I have since come to the conclusion that inactivity is a first-class phantom enabler. Gradually, I got back into a regular daily routine. I caught up with my professional continuing education requirements, and I exercised again. Stepping up the activity felt good.

While keeping busy is fine, it is also important to guard against becoming manic. Some people put themselves into a continuous, frenzied activity mode in an effort to escape their tinnitus annoyance. A woman mentioned in a group meeting that she "tried so hard" to ignore the noises all day that she ran herself ragged. In the evening she was exhausted and stressed out, her tinnitus was raging, and then she had trouble sleeping. Yet she was sure that her best tinnitus antidote was her "mind over matter" approach.

Learning how to take the noise out of tinnitus is much more than "mind over matter." As the doctor pointed out in his speech, tinnitus habituation is a process that happens slowly, over time, on a *subconscious* level. It comes from within. Mind over matter deals with the conscious mind, in the now, and does not recalibrate our negative bias. Obviously, it did not work very well for this lady. She seemed to spend a major portion of her day feeding adrenaline to known tinnitus triggers.

Thinking of Others while Remembering the Self

After my ear event, I spent some time in a funk, but I gradually picked up life where I had left off. I also began to think about others, which added a new dimension to my hearing loss and tinnitus mayhem. I had taken those who cared about me for granted. I also realized that living with me was not exactly an easy task anymore. Yes, I needed to make some adjustments in my attitude toward the phantom, but I also had to make a serious course correction as far as my family and friends were concerned. This was when I joined two support groups. I began to care deeply about my brethren, many of whom had a much harder lot than mine. As I turned my attention away from myself and from the hissing and got involved with other people and projects, the noises became more tolerable.

Dealing with tinnitus is a challenge that takes energy and motivation. While it is important to be engaged with family and social matters, it is equally important not to forget about ourselves. We are supposed to draw on our inner strengths for healing, yet now and then, that inner well must also be replenished. I have never been one for spending much time relaxing or indulging in something that I enjoyed. Now, thanks to the phantom, I give myself more time for that. As I love history and documentaries, I treat myself to the occasional good book or movie. And a massage with lavender oil? Now we are talking.

Rediscovering a Sense of Humor

I recently saw a rerun of *Seinfeld,* in which Uncle Leo had ringing in the ears. "Sounds like the phone," he said. At some point, becoming frustrated, he yelled at the patrons in the coffee shop if anyone was ever going to answer that darn phone. I strongly identified with him, even though I "hear" something so different. I actually laughed because it struck me as a funny in-joke. Had I seen this episode a few years ago, when I was in the initial throes of hearing loss and of being driven crazy by tinnitus, I probably would have been furious. It was great to know that my sense of humor was waking up—an unmistakable sign of improvement.

***

A Work in Progress

Tinnitus has taught me something that I never had: patience. It reminds me daily that I am signed up for the long haul. Although I practice focus-shifting and relaxation techniques on a regular basis, my sometimes hesitant and still inconsistent efforts at retraining my brain are ongoing. Sometimes, I am taken by surprise and respond with intolerance to the phantom. It might be a brief experience, but it proves that I have not totally succeeded in internalizing some of the de-conditioning tactics; they have not yet become second nature to me, and I am still learning.

As my tinnitus shifts around a lot, it can prove difficult to be in an emotionally neutral state at all times. However, I taught both myself and my brain a few new tricks over time. Overall, the noises have become less aggressive, and that is a most welcome change. I do believe that as I tame myself, I also tame the ear din. I use my noise-reducing headset with the nature tunes a lot less frequently than I used to do. The phantom does not monopolize my attention every minute of the day anymore, which has made our co-existence a lot more peaceful.

Thanks to the massive incentive that tinnitus provided, my life became more balanced than it had been for a while. Yet maintaining that balance continues to be a bit of an issue due to my somewhat Type-A personality. Every day is a new beginning and often also a new challenge.

In the end, the truth is that—as I got out of the funk—both my productivity and self-image perked up. Right now, I have left the box canyon of tinnitus behind and continue on the path that widens in front of me. I definitely remain optimistic, while also managing my expectations.

Chapter 27
Professional Tinnitus Management:
Products, Treatments, Medications

Most tinnitus patients have their own secret ways for dealing with the noises. In our support group meetings, we share our successes and failures. Yet homespun recipes often are not enough and can be inappropriate and even counterproductive. So it is important to recognize one's limits. Novice tinnitus sufferers, those who have had poor results with home-style therapy, and those whose lives are turned upside down by the phantom all should take solace in the fact that professional help is available.

The point has already been made that people with ear or head noises should get checked by an ear specialist. The best outcome would be to get rid of the sounds altogether. If it is not possible, however, to silence the clamor by eliminating its cause, help is available from various sources—specialized physicians, audiologists, therapists, and the hearing industry. Getting relief from tinnitus that is *not* related to a treatable condition is essentially a trial-and-error approach. There is no single good answer; what works for one person does not necessarily work another. Yet devices and treatment techniques offered by hearing experts, such as audiologists, might ease the annoyance. Specialized tinnitus clinics also are there to assist.

Hearing Aids and Tinnitus Relief
Those whose tinnitus is due to hearing loss might benefit from the use of a hearing aid. No matter how sophisticated they are, hearing aids are basically sound amplifiers. Often, people become less aware of their ear noises when their world is made less silent by the hearing instrument. If the tinnitus is not too loud, an increase in overall sound

volume can hide the noise and give the patient some relief. It is also hoped that an acceptable amount of amplification across the hearing loss frequencies might restore enough signal transmission to convince the brain to give up or to ease its search for input. Of course, once the hearing aid is removed, the noises are again audible, yet even a few hours of daily peace could make a huge difference in a patient's quality of life.

Although hearing aids do not "cure" tinnitus, they can help in certain cases, depending on the type and extent of the hearing loss, and are worth a try. However, it takes a skilled and patient hearing specialist to figure out which hearing device features are best suited to help a tinnitus client.

Some manufacturers incorporate tinnitus-managing sound programs into their instruments. Lately, wind-chime-like tones, referred to as *fractal sounds*, are a new approach to soothing the tinnitus annoyance. Unfortunately, hearing aids—with or without built-in sound therapy—have *not* performed magic tricks on my tinnitus, although various audiologists have tried to give me a break from the din by manipulating my device. For me, louder was definitely not better, and there were points beyond which the phantom got quite irritated.

As every case of hearing loss is different, so is every case of tinnitus. The important thing is to be aware of the many available features that might bring relief and to ask about them. When I was first fitted for a hearing instrument, I was not knowledgeable enough to ask questions. I was unaware that hearing instruments even had the potential to relieve tinnitus under the right circumstances. However, I have since met people who credit their hearing aids for getting some peace back into their lives, which is a wonderful thing.

Masking the Phantom

Masking is a technique for covering up internal sounds, tinnitus, with external sounds, or masking sounds. The ear noises are "masked" as they lose themselves within the outside noises. Eventually, the brain learns to *ignore* the masking sound and with it, the tinnitus. If the strategy works, the ear din becomes less noticeable or even unnoticeable. As the sound sources are used whenever the patient needs relief, masking offers flexible control over the tinnitus annoyance.

Masking is often suggested as an intervention for those whose noises are excessively distressing or debilitating. It works best for clients who have little or no hearing loss because the brain must be able to perceive the masking sounds. Patients with hearing loss might be able to detect masking noises only if they wear their hearing aids. Although it can be helpful, masking is not perfect. It has its limits for patients with fluctuating tinnitus, for those whose tinnitus incorporates several different tones, or for those with a pronounced hearing loss. In these cases, the help of a savvy audiologist is needed for easing the ear phantom.

The generic approach to tinnitus masking typically involves white noise—static from off-the-air radio or TV stations, high-speed fans, and running water of faucets and showers. White noise can be used by itself or, more pleasantly, it can be incorporated with other soothing, more melodious themes that are relaxing for the patient. An added masking benefit might be that tinnitus abatement continues even after the masking sounds stop. This is referred to as "residual inhibition," which can last from minutes to hours and maybe longer.

187

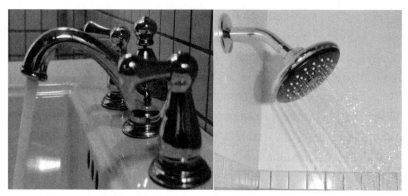

Many people report that running water can help mask their tinnitus.
photo: R.Hammond

Running water sounds are known to be the most effective tinnitus maskers. People mention frequently that their ear noises seem much relieved and almost neutralized when they are in the shower. As the tinnitus blends with the frequency-rich white noise produced by the running water, the phantom's antics become less evident. Besides the shower effect, a simple way to get an idea if masking might help is to take the "faucet test." Turn on the water taps full blast, and lean the tinnitus ear toward the sound produced by the rushing water. If the tinnitus is no longer detectable, there is a good chance that masking could be of benefit.

During the faucet test, I sense an overall lessening of the noise, but the bothersome very high pitches are still there. Within the gushing water sounds, I simply do not 'hear" those frequencies that would help cover up or counteract the corresponding high frequencies of my tinnitus.

Masking Products

Commercially available CDs or online programs and apps offer frequency mixes that have the best potential to wrap themselves around the tinnitus noise, mingle with it, cover it up, or neutralize it. Usually, the masking sounds are incorporated into tunes that help to distract and relax, which are important features in tinnitus management. Audiologists sell commercially made tinnitus *distracter/masker* units. These are sound generators, not sound amplifiers. They are the size of hearing aids and are worn like them. The devices are pre-programmed with plain white noise, with or without music. They also can be custom-programmed by the audiologist with masking sound mixes that work best for the client. People might prefer the masker option because the small devices can be worn unobtrusively anywhere and unlike a CD, they play without interruption.

Wearable units are also available for people with hearing loss whose tinnitus is not helped by a hearing aid. Referred to as *tinnitus instruments*, dual or combination devices are dispensed by hearing specialists. They combine the hearing aid function with a masking-sound generator.

To find out if a wearable tinnitus masker is appropriate or which brand has the best features, we should rely on our audiologist's opinion. Also, as these devices can be pricey, we must ask about the trial period, warranties, refund policies, and payment arrangements before we buy, just as we do when purchasing a hearing aid.

Matching and Masking

Commercially available generic masking sounds can be quite effective, but audiologists now have the ability to custom-design a masking base that *matches* the patient's tinnitus pattern. Although silence is not guaranteed, this could be worth a try. Assisted by special computer software, the hearing expert identifies the frequencies, overall tone, and intensity of the tinnitus. The resulting signal can be further blended with calming music for a more acceptable listening experience. The mix is programmed onto a CD or a masker unit or it might be transferred to an MP3 player or smartphone, which might be a more affordable option. When tinnitus tests their resilience, people listen to this sound and lull the phantom to sleep. In essence, matching the tinnitus noise makes masking more specific and, therefore, more effective. The ear noises are washed out or neutralized. Of course, the hoped-for side effect of the treatment is that of a possible residual inhibition, but there is no way of telling if this might happen.

***

The expressions noise "cover-up" or "masking" can be misleading. As I found out, there are those who get carried away with their efforts not to "hear" the annoying ear noises anymore. They crank the volume of the MP3 player to the max in an attempt to obliterate the tinnitus with all sorts of music, including rock and heavy metal that is way too loud. Frustration runs high when the phantom becomes even more aggressive in response to the decibel barrage. As expected, exciting the brain further pushes the tinnitus intensity in the wrong direction. More importantly, exaggerated noise levels damage hearing, and we know that hearing damage begets more tinnitus. Instead, the use of a calming mix of tinnitus-wrapping sounds might well convince the brain to downshift its frenetic activity and grant a reprieve from the clatter.

PSTR Tinnitus Treatment

PSTR stands for phase-shift tinnitus reduction. This technique applies to tinnitus that presents as a *single* frequency sound. After passing an initial physical evaluation and qualifying as a candidate, the client's tinnitus signal is "sound-typed" for studying and matching of its specific frequency and loudness pattern. By means of highly technical equipment, the exact tinnitus signal is then reproduced and gradually "phase-shifted." This means that a signal of *equal but opposite* quality to the original tinnitus noise is eventually created. That manipulated signal, which cancels out the original tinnitus signal, is presented to the patient through headphones during treatments at the

190

clinic. If effective, the phase-shifted sound pattern is transferred to a special device for home-use. Obviously, the secret lies in the absolutely exact match of the tinnitus sound wave. The signal is rechecked at regular intervals to make sure that the tinnitus frequency has not changed. If this has happened, the device must be reprogrammed. It is said that residual inhibition can last on average a week or longer for patients who have been successfully treated with this technique.

Ultrasound Treatment

Devices that use ultrasound energy for tinnitus management are another option that can be discussed with the audiologist. The target area for treatment is the mastoid bone behind the ear. Usually handheld, these appliances are prescribed by a physician or audiologist and can be tested in the office. The dispensing practitioner will explain the rationale for using ultrasound to counteract tinnitus, what can be expected from the treatment and instruct the client in the correct use and function of the instrument.

It is important to get information about limiting side effects, manufacturer warnings, precautions, contraindications, and care instructions. Once more, it is good to inquire about trial periods, instrument warranty, and cost details.

Repetitive Transcranial Magnetic Stimulation (rTMS)

In the case of tinnitus, the purpose of rTMS would be to calm overly active hearing structures in the brain by means of magnetic energy pulses. In theory, less activity should translate into less ear and head noise. However, clinical trials have been small and results have been erratic. rTMS is reported to have eased tinnitus perception in some study patients, but its effects are inconsistent. Besides, researchers are not sure of its exact mechanism in tinnitus, and the procedure is not without possible side effects or complications. Larger and longer trials, together with revisions of research protocols, might lead to clearer insights in the future. rTMS is currently not FDA-approved for tinnitus.

***

Obviously, there are quite a few ways to potentially reduce tinnitus annoyance. Before falling prey to advertising gimmicks, it is best to have an honest tinnitus-reduction talk with a hearing expert. Professionals have the most practical experience and up-to-date information on tinnitus-taming techniques and devices. I have found hearing specialists to be sensitive to my cost concerns and willing to provide feedback on self-help techniques and commercial products. Asking for advice will keep us from making uninformed and misguided decisions that could make our condition worse. After all, our aim is to coax the phantom back into its box, not to cause it to throw ever more aggressive tantrums.

***

Professionally Guided Therapies

Various therapeutic strategies can be used to provide long-term relief for tinnitus suffers. These work mostly on our inner core—our emotions, beliefs, attitudes, and reactions. They are not cures or quick-and-easy fixes, and our commitment is needed for these approaches to be successful. Although they do not come with any guarantees, they can help us regain control over ourselves and our lives.

So far, I have not attended any formal programs, but I also have not excluded them. They figure among my fallback plans, should I have to wage a serious battle on the phantom in the future.

Cognitive-behavioral Therapy (CBT)

Cognitive-behavioral therapy recognizes the fact that our thoughts play an important role in how we act and how we feel. Although CBT can be used to treat many different problems, the underlying principles have been helpful when counseling tinnitus patients who are trying to deal with their ear ruckus. CBT teaches how to change or adjust our thinking process on a particular issue—in this case, tinnitus. CBT might help us escape the distress caused by distorted thoughts and perceptions that we harbor against our condition and which end up affecting our quality of life.

There are several ways for talking ourselves into a slump. We exaggerate things. We over-generalize. We dwell on the negative. We jump to conclusions that emphasize the dismal. Eventually, our negative emotions and reactions become our reality.

Once we are caught in the downward spiral of tension, stress, and desperation, it is often hard to turn around on our own. In order to break the cycle that feeds the ear noise, we might consider consulting with a CBT specialist. These counselors help clients analyze their condition as well as their reactions to it. They do not tell them what to do or how they should feel. Instead, by using different techniques and concepts, they *teach* how to substitute accurate and realistic thoughts for the negative, counterproductive ones. Once people learn how to think and react differently, they can build on that experience.

CBT is not never-ending talk therapy. It is an educational process, a collaboration that involves the counselor and the client. Sessions are structured and focused and involve homework. In order to get the most out of the meetings, a good working relationship between client and therapist is a must, as is the client's commitment to the program. The National Association of Cognitive-Behavioral Therapists (NACBT) states that CBT is a briefer, time-limited therapy that runs, on average, sixteen sessions.

Sound Therapy and Directive Counseling

The combination of sound therapy and directive counseling form the basis of two professional programs that are said to have the best chance to help tinnitus sufferers curb the noise annoyance for good: *TRT* and *Neuromonics*. At the end of the treatment, the phantom is still there but it is no longer important in our lives.

One might wonder why all tinnitus sufferers are not all enrolled in such a program. Through my totally unscientific, grassroots survey, I found out that a fair number of people did not know about these options. Others had heard about them but did not know any details. Those who did know had four major reasons for passing on the therapies: they are lengthy, costly, offer no guarantees for success, and the noise will not be gone. Obviously, misunderstandings regarding the purpose of these treatments and the notion of "success" keep lingering. There are those, however, who feel that their therapy was a godsend and time and money well-spent.

Professional tinnitus treatment programs are administered by *specially trained practitioners* who will teach, counsel, and guide the clients. A positive outcome depends to a large extent on the patient's readiness to commit to the plan and on his/her ability to work with the assigned specialist. If the patient and the counselor are incompatible, it is better to ask for someone else rather than abandon the whole program.

As *costs* are a major concern, however, it is important to ask about them up front. Clinics with high overhead expenses, such as those in prime locations or with extra staff, do charge more. We are well advised to ask for a breakdown of the charges, such as the initial consult/screening session, extra hearing evaluations, the sound device, the actual counseling, any extra counseling sessions, and the follow-up care. We also need details regarding payment plans, deposits, refund policies, instrument warranties, and any extra charges. We also should inquire about possible insurance coverage. A referral certificate from the physician might be needed for the insurance to help with at least some of the charges.

Because these therapies rely on the expertise of specially trained clinicians, it is perfectly fine to ask about their *credentials,* where they were trained, and how long they have worked with the program.

To avoid surprises, we should inquire about the counselor's task and clarify how often we will meet with him/her, how long the sessions will last, and how the counseling will be delivered: face-to-face, by telephone, or by e-mail. Then, if we decide to try one of these treatments, we must be ready to give it our best shot and to accept the costs. In the end, if it works for us, it will have been worth every penny.

Tinnitus Retraining Therapy (TRT)

Tinnitus retraining therapy is a professionally guided habituation program that was developed by Dr. Pawel J. Jastreboff and has been available since the 1990s. The treatment goal is to make tinnitus irrelevant in our lives—it might still be there, but it is no longer meaningful. Before accepting patients into the program, the clinic will make sure that the necessary, preliminary hearing and medical checks have been completed.

TRT involves low-level broadband *noise* and *"directive counseling"* provided by practitioners who are specially trained in the elements that make up TRT.

Directive counseling is a must—it is a cornerstone of the therapy. It consists of a series of intense, interactive educational sessions. Patients learn the details of how the tinnitus noises insert themselves into their lives. They are taught how the auditory system interacts with important other areas of the nervous system, such as the limbic (emotional) and autonomic (fight-or-flight) centers. Targeted education helps the clients disengage these systems as far as tinnitus is concerned. In essence, the brain must learn to block the tinnitus signal from reaching these areas and from interacting with them.

The main purpose of directive counseling is to demystify the phantom and to yank the patients out of the trap of erroneous beliefs and negative attitudes that influence their behavior toward the noise. In the end, the din in their ears is no longer fed by contrary emotions and anxiety-plagued reactions. Tinnitus leaves them neutral.

Besides the teaching component, counselors also monitor the client's progress and provide instructions on special retraining exercises. In return, the patient must be able to absorb and digest the material and follow the directions provided by the specialist. Usually, there is an initial directive counseling session, followed by two or three more over the time of the treatment period, which lasts on average twelve to eighteen months. As the patient and the counselor work together, it is expected that the tinnitus annoyance will gradually lessen. Although the signal still will be there, it is not "heard" unless the patient tunes into it or seeks it.

Tinnitus sufferers know that total silence allows the phantom to squawk even louder. Therefore, during the course of TRT therapy, clients must *avoid total silence* twenty-four hours a day; this is a core therapy requirement. The environment needs to be sound-enriched rather than deathly still, so patients are instructed to listen to calming, pleasant music or to white noise at all times.

The sounds, however, must be at a low enough level *not* to mask or cover the ear noise. The tinnitus signal must remain detectable by the brain. The rationale is that the brain cannot habituate itself or get used to noises that are continuously cloaked. During treatment, patients also wear broadband noise generators that are designed and adjusted to help with the habituation process. TRT accommodates people with hearing loss as they can use "tinnitus instruments," the hearing aid/sound generator combination units mentioned earlier, during therapy.

A major ingredient for TRT success is the rapport that exists between the patient and the directive counselor. There may be, however, a tendency to misunderstand or misinterpret the TRT notion of "counseling."

TRT counselors have a different role from the traditional counselor, who is more a listener and confidant. In TRT, the counselors act as teachers and mentors. Of course, they have compassion for their clients, but they do not want them to dwell on the annoyance aspect of tinnitus. Their primary purpose is to convey information to the patient, together with suggestions on how to apply what is learned to their life. Figuratively speaking, TRT counselors "direct" the focus away from tinnitus suffering.

Neuromonics

Neuromonics is a newer sound-counseling approach for tinnitus treatment. Developed by audiologist Dr. Paul Davis, Neuromonics comes to us from Australia. Here, too, the purpose is to reduce the negative impact that tinnitus has on clients' lives and to render them tinnitus-neutral. The mainstays of the Neuromonics program are sound therapy combined with "directive counseling." It takes on average six to eight months to complete the treatment.

For my personal understanding, I translate "Neuromonics" loosely as "brain-tuning music." As "music" is indeed at the center of the therapy, it is important to be able to "hear" the music. Although people with hearing loss might be at a disadvantage, the specially trained audiologist decides if they are candidates for the therapy. The treatment sound is delivered to the patient through specially designed headphones by the Neuromonics FDA-approved processor (about the size of an MP3 player), appropriately named "Oasis."

After the patient has had a thorough medical check-up, the next step is to perform a comprehensive set of hearing tests and tinnitus evaluations. This is most important because the Oasis will be programmed by the company with an acoustic signal that is modified and customized, according to the patient's tinnitus and hearing profiles. The time from the initial visit to receiving delivery of the custom-programmed device is about two weeks.

The individualized, music pattern is designed to retrain and reprogram the brain to filter out the tinnitus noise. It also helps to relax the patient and takes the mind off the tinnitus annoyance. People with fluctuating, complex, or changing tinnitus sounds might not be the best candidates for this program. It takes a specialist who is intimately familiar with the treatment criteria and protocol to successfully screen clients and advise them whether Neuromonics might be helpful.

The Neuromonics sound treatment is delivered in two stages. Stage I typically lasts for the first two months. The immediate purpose is to relieve the tinnitus symptoms and to give the patient a feeling of control over the phantom. During this stage, white noise is embedded in the music blend, which allows for some tinnitus masking. The patient listens on average two to four hours per day to the therapy sound, not necessarily all at once. It is best to listen while in a relaxed state so that the brain-retraining tunes are allowed to soak in. Some patients schedule their sessions, or parts of them, while they eat quietly, read a book, go for a leisurely walk, or before they go to bed.

Flexibility, a pleasant listening experience, and a potentially fast response have contributed to Neuromonics's gain in popularity. The company mentions that it takes anywhere from one to thirty days for people to notice relief.

Stage II takes up the next four months. This active treatment phase is meant to break the tinnitus cycle. Now the brain actually learns to filter out the tinnitus signal. The Oasis sound is adjusted to let the tinnitus noise break intermittently through the music. Since the client is used to listening to the music, he/she does not concentrate on the tinnitus. It is simply another noise that is ignored. The patient listens for at least two hours a day to the device. As desensitization occurs, treatment times are gradually reduced. Once the patient has successfully completed the program, the specialized clinician will help him/her develop a self-help maintenance program to preserve the benefits derived from treatment.

It is important for patients to know that sound treatment is only part of the whole protocol and the role of directive counseling must not be ignored. In Neuromonics, the counselor is also a teacher and mentor who familiarizes the client with the emotional and physical details of tinnitus. The counselor also monitors the patient's treatment compliance and progress. In short, the Oasis device cannot do it all. A clinic that downplays or skips directive counseling deprives the patient of a key portion of the treatment plan, and it pays to search for a better fit.

Tinnitus Management and Medications

If tinnitus is not due to an underlying cause that can be fixed or treated, we are left to deal with the mysterious subjective ear and head noises that seem to come out of nowhere. Yet identifying and managing any aggravating factors, such as allergies, sinus problems, or chronic ear wax issues, can already make quite a difference. Any little bit helps.

So far, no medications are approved by the FDA for treating tinnitus specifically. Drugs aimed at alleviating symptoms might help in some cases but not in others. Everyone's ear phantom is up to different tricks, which presents scientists with a variety of challenges. Although it is encouraging to know that the search for a tinnitus-silencing agent is going on worldwide, it will be a while before the noises can be squelched effectively and predictably by medication.

Now and then my hopes get raised by the appearance of articles that report on a substance that shows "promise" for tinnitus noise suppression, but so far we do not have any clear winners. Following up on current tinnitus theories, researchers have tested many existing medications and chemicals, only to be frustrated by often disappointing results. With every trial, however, new insights are gained. It could be that the drug that liberates us from the noises is one that we already know, one that has been sitting on the shelf all this time. Then again, it could be that the tinnitus-busting substance has not been invented yet. Researchers might be forced to develop brand new compounds as they close in on the nervous pathways hijacked by the phantom.

As I have been reminded so often on this journey, time will tell. As I already noted, the first trip for people with ear or head noise should be to a specialist for a physical exam and hearing evaluations. Drug management for tinnitus depends a lot on the type of tinnitus. It takes a devoted and astute physician to become wise to the ear noises, to order the most relevant tests, and to formulate a diagnosis. Patients with telltale pulsatile tinnitus noises are often referred to internists and other specialists for care. The following discussion focuses on some of the medicines that can make subjective tinnitus less of a challenge.

Because subjective tinnitus might be a symptom of quite a few underlying conditions, the physician is faced with a brand new search for each patient. If the root cause for the ear noises cannot be found and eliminated, it is often quite helpful to manage triggers and aggravating factors. Any bit that can be shaved off the annoyance is worth the effort. As patients, we rely heavily on the expertise of our tinnitus physicians who advise us if management with medications is possible.

I appreciated the candor of my specialist, who told me that there was no medication available to soothe my ear clamor directly—a harsh but honest assessment. I actually am not keen on attacking the noises generically with hard-hitting drugs that often have many side effects and produce questionable results. For now, I am able to manage without medication. I will continue, however, to hone my skills at disengaging the emotional input that feeds the phantom and count on the miracles from within.

Medications Tried for Tinnitus Relief

In their endeavors to minimize symptoms, doctors use various agents to bring relief to tinnitus patients. The following general discussion focuses on some of the commonly used medicines. It is important to remember that the medications mentioned in this section are *not specific* for tinnitus and are used according to special protocols for treating many different conditions. Their use is mentioned here *in the context of tinnitus only.* Patients who are being treated with these drugs for whatever reason must follow their doctors' orders and guidance and refer any questions or concerns that might arise from this account to their specialist or pharmacist.

The menu of medicines that have been tried for tinnitus relief features anti-anxiety, anti-panic, and antidepressant medications, among others. Amazingly, some agents that are meant to bring tinnitus relief also figure on the lists of drugs suspected of causing it. This proves once more that not all ear noises are created equal, and that the physician's experience, wise judgment, and patient-counseling skills are more critical than ever.

Benzodiazepines, or "Benzos"

Currently, no medications are FDA-approved for treating tinnitus, which includes the benzodiazepines. Although they remain quite popular, these are powerful medicines that affect brain, mind, and body. Different members of this large family have their own special features and indications. Usage and dosing guidelines depend largely on the diagnosis, condition, and age of the patient and the properties of the drug.

The benzodiazepines include medications for treating multiple conditions, such as anxiety, panic, tension, muscle spasticity, certain seizures, and insomnia. As vestibular suppressants, they can also help with dizziness and balance issues, an effect that is particularly helpful in patients with Ménière's disease. Benzodiazepines are, however, *controlled substances* that must be *closely monitored by the prescriber.* Unless they are deliberately abused, they are considered relatively safe, if taken at appropriate doses for short periods of time. They are said to have low addiction potential, which does *not* mean that they don't have any addiction potential. There is a troubling aspect to these medications. Getting on them is easy. The issue often becomes how to get off. We must ask about that ahead of time.

201

Certainly, ever since their appearance on the medical scene, the benzodiazepines—of which diazepam (*Valium*) is the granddaddy—have helped many people over rough spots in life. In the world of hearing loss, tinnitus, and Ménière's disease, the use, benefits, and pitfalls of these agents tend to stir up controversy among specialists and patients alike. Frequently encountered members of this family are alprazolam (*Xanax*), clonazepam (*Klonopin*), diazepam (*Valium*), lorazepam (*Ativan*), and oxazepam (*Serax*).

In support groups, I have come across a fair number of people who are or who have been on a benzodiazepine or two. Among group attendees, just about every one of the different agents in this drug class is represented and has its supporters and detractors. The answers to the question of how well they work are as spotty as the reports from the professional community. However, people mostly agree that their overall calming effect is quite beneficial for tinnitus and Ménière's management and that the occasional use of a benzodiazepine can spell relief in trying times when all else seems to fail.

Although the use of these drugs is widespread in our rather stressed-out, anxious midst, there are some common truths about them that we should be aware of, so that we can discuss them up front with the doctor. Once we start treatment with these agents, continued good communication with the prescriber is of the essence. It is important that we understand how they fit into our overall treatment plan—why they are used, when they should be used, and for how long they can be used.

Benzodiazepines act relatively quickly—a plus for people who are in acute distress. They do not "cure" tinnitus. They mostly ease the panic, tension, and anxiety that are often associated with tinnitus and can make it worse. They help the patient relax and maybe get some much-needed sleep. They blunt our reaction to the ear din, which is much easier to tolerate once we settle down a bit. Drowsiness is, of course, one of the first benzodiazepine side effects. If we are helped by the medication, we should take that as an indicator that life with the ear phantom is possible and become inspired to check on other long-term management strategies with the physician or audiologist.

Although they buy us time, benzodiazepines are generally not meant to be taken in high dosages, long term, on a regular daily basis, *unless* we are specifically instructed to do so under the very watchful eye of the physician who has a specific goal in mind. Even then, patients must be aware of those circumstances that dictate when to get in touch with the doctor most urgently. The problem is that with uninterrupted use, these medicines will gradually lose their effect, which is a major reason why they do not offer a daily, long-term solution for us. However, when taken intermittently, on an "as needed" basis, or for short periods of time, they can remain effective longer.

Need for Clarification of Prescription Instructions

In order to provide relief during a rough spell, the specialist often allows for some short-term, regular daily dosing. It is important, however, for the doctor to discuss the time frame for "short term" with us. Does this mean days, weeks, or months? We must be clear on the doctor's intent as the definition for short term depends on the medication, the diagnosis, and the patients' ability to metabolize and eliminate the drug.

For our purposes, prescription labels usually carry the instructions to take the prescribed doses "as needed". This concept opens a window for misinterpretation and must also be explained to patients. What defines a "need," and how long should that "need" be allowed to continue before we must call for additional guidance on the issue?

Generally, "as needed" means that the medication serves as a rescue on difficult days when the ear noise is particularly annoying or anxiety-provoking. One might think of stress events that kick the phantom into gear.

Although the medicine is ordered "as needed," some patients end up taking it at maximum allowed doses, day after day after day. They figure that they "need" the drug continuously because the ear noises bother them continuously. Pretty soon they venture out onto the slippery slope of daily, long-term use. "Needing the drug all the time" calls for a discussion with the physician on what the agent can and cannot do for them. The concern is that people expect the medication to carry the full load, postpone dealing with the realities of their condition, and neglect making necessary lifestyle changes.

The Tolerance and Dependence Traps

Daily, chronic use, especially at high doses, leads to benzodiazepine tolerance and dependence. *Tolerance* means that the drugs lose their effectiveness at the prescribed dose. In order to get the same results, the body requests more medication. This is a warning sign that a new management plan is urgently needed. Whenever it feels that the medicine does not work as well as it once did, it is essential to have a serious discussion with the prescriber regarding long-term tolerance problems and the need for a new strategy.

Tolerance brings us to a crossroads, and action must be taken. The decision might be to increase the dosage of the first drug, to add a second benzodiazepine, or to change to a different agent within the same drug class. Predictably, after continuous use, the new drug regimen leads right back to tolerance. It is easy to see how one could wind up in a frustrating escalation trap. Rather than insisting on dosage adjustments or trying different benzodiazepines, alone or in combination, one should question if it would be wiser to wean the benzodiazepine(s) *ever so slowly* under medical supervision and to look into an alternative plan altogether. These are the important decisions that face both the physician and patient.

Uninterrupted, daily benzodiazepine use also can lead to *physical dependence*. The hallmark of physical dependence is the appearance of withdrawal symptoms, especially if the medication is stopped abruptly or if there is a sudden decrease in dosage. Often, those who have taken the medicine regularly are not aware that they have become physically dependent on it until they forget to take a dose or delay taking the medication. They might have little explanation for mysterious symptoms that suddenly beset them and do not suspect their medication as a possible cause. However, breakthrough withdrawal signs may occur even while the patient takes the drug regularly at prescribed dosages.

The list of possible benzodiazepine withdrawal symptoms is varied and lengthy. Patients may report having digestive problems, cramping, nausea, lack of appetite, insomnia, muscle cramps, and headaches. Anxiety and panic reactions also have been described. Tinnitus that had become bearable might be back with a vengeance. Heart palpitations and heart pounding are mentioned, as are being antsy, agitated, lightheaded, and impatient. Benzodiazepine withdrawal can lead to an altered sense of sound. Sounds may seem louder, tinny or distorted. Amazingly enough *tinnitus* itself also appears on the long, long list of known withdrawal symptoms for these drugs.

Once more, the body signals in so many ways that an urgent treatment revision is needed. Now, the patient *must* talk to the doctor at once and ask for advice on how to proceed. Until that time, the dose should not be altered. Making sudden changes, or worse yet, stopping the medication abruptly after long term use, could have serious and even dangerous consequences, such as anxiety reactions and seizures that require a trip to the emergency room. Instead, the doctor must make the necessary recommendations for dealing with the issue. Tolerance and physical dependence mark tough times for both the patient and the physician.

Along with signs of physical dependence, symptoms of *psychological* dependence eventually emerge; patients do not want to give up the medication even though it has lost its effectiveness and now causes them other problems and more harm than good. In some ways, people grow afraid of life without the drug. They might doctor-shop, purchase the medication online, and exhibit different levels of drug-seeking behaviors. Any excuse for remaining on the medication seems like a good excuse.

The way to get off benzodiazepines, especially once tolerance and dependence of any kind set in, is to *taper* the dosage down very, very gradually over time under the direction of a knowledgeable physician. Weaning off these drugs is a *slow* process and not a do-it-yourself endeavor. Going too fast or quitting "cold turkey" throws the brain chemistry into disarray, which can be quite unpleasant and even dangerous. It might be necessary to get a *referral* to a competent rehab specialist who can manage a benzodiazepine tapering/weaning program while supporting and monitoring the patient during the process.

***

Benzodiazepines can be quite helpful to tinnitus and Ménière's patients, yet it is important not to underestimate the power of these agents. If a benzodiazepine is prescribed, we must discuss the positives and negatives of the drug with the doctor. We might inquire about the physician's experience with a particular agent in a case such as ours. We want to clarify the prescription instructions, what types of symptoms will indicate that tolerance or dependence might become issues and what actions we should then take. It is also to our advantage to read and understand the patient information that comes with the prescription as these medications have many side effects, precautions, and warnings. Most of all, we must realize that medications can only help so much, and that it is always wise to check on alternate tinnitus-taming strategies as early as possible.

***

Antidepressants

Many patients with tinnitus, especially chronic tinnitus, also suffer from depression. If this is found to be the case, the doctor might consider using an antidepressant drug in order to calm the ear din, although not all patients respond to this type of treatment. The tangled emotional web that the phantom can spin presents the specialist with some unique challenges. While listening to a patient's story, the physician must clarify if the tinnitus causes the depression or if the depression causes or worsens the tinnitus. He/she will also scan for underlying signs of panic, anxiety, or even obsession that keeps the clients fixated on the phantom, which, of course, gives it a tremendous amount of power over their lives.

Although there are different classes of antidepressants, doctors usually resort to the newer SSRIs (selective serotonin reuptake inhibitors). The agents in this group increase the brain levels of serotonin, one of the substances that play an important role in depression. Depending on their unique chemical structures, however, different members of the SSRI family can also help with aggravating factors that go beyond depression, such as panic, anxiety, and obsessive-compulsive behaviors. Guided by our emotional symptoms, the doctor will choose the most appropriate medication.

There is no sure way of predicting how our ear phantom will react to an antidepressant, and therapy may proceed by trial and error. Because tinnitus is listed as a possible side effect for a number of these drugs, different medications might have to be tried before finding one that is acceptable.

To be sure, antidepressants are no quick fixes; it usually takes a few weeks before they begin to work. It is important to discuss the onset lag with the doctor so that we know what to expect. SSRIs should not be stopped abruptly. Dosages are gradually tapered up or down *under the strict supervision of the prescriber*. Also, antidepressants are certainly not without their warnings and precautions, and we must review those up front with the physician. For example, patients are warned to report any worsening of their depression and/or suicidal thoughts to their doctor at once.

That said, for people who have both tinnitus and depression, it is essential to discuss the situation with the doctor. If there is a chance that an antidepressant might reduce the ear din and make life easier, it could be worth a try. As we say in the world of tinnitus, any little bit helps.

More Options

Before medicating ourselves with various advertised and other over-the-counter products, we must not forget that tinnitus is a *symptom* that has to be evaluated by a medical specialist for reasons already amply discussed.

As far as tinnitus is concerned, there is not much in this world that has not been tried in order to gain some peace. It is often hard to figure out if there is any reasonable science behind the touted tinnitus-relief products, what their downsides might be, or how they will interact with other medications that we may be taking.

Yet for every product, there are those who claim relief. We all react differently to pharmaceuticals, and our own convictions and beliefs can be our biggest allies. Because there are no accredited studies to guide us, testimonials from happy customers become usually the only source of "information."

Tinnitus-relief formulas are often *homeopathic* in nature. They are composed of multiple ingredients that are present in tiny amounts. All we have to go on are the manufacturer's guidelines for dosing and the length of treatment before results might be expected.

Vitamin and mineral supplements formulated for tinnitus sufferers are also quite popular. If the noises are due to a true underlying deficiency, they can be of help. Deficiencies in certain vitamins, notably vitamin B-12, and minerals such as zinc have been tied to some tinnitus cases. Although these products are available over-the-counter, they have precautions just like any other medication does. Before taking extra supplements, we'd best confer first with the doctor. Maybe our actual blood levels should be checked before we load up on things that we might not even need.

Gingko biloba is often highly advertised as a tinnitus remedy and is an ingredient in many relief recipes. Its antioxidant properties give the herb qualities that could have positive ear effects. However, overall study results on gingko's tinnitus-busting capabilities are often contradictory. Yet there are those who claim that they tried it and it helped. It all depends on the case, but ginkgo has its definite advocates. Dosage recommendations for tinnitus treatment are inconsistent, and some are on the high side.

In Europe the herb is recommended for tinnitus associated with hearing loss, especially if a vascular or blood circulation component is suspected. Poor circulation and therefore low oxygen levels in the ear are often cited as contributing to both hearing loss and tinnitus. In these cases, the use of ginkgo would make sense. It thins the blood and increases blood flow by dilating blood vessels, which, in theory, leads to improved inner-ear oxygen levels and, hopefully, tinnitus abatement. For whatever reason, the ear noise often does not respond. Maybe there is no blood supply issue connected with the tinnitus.

The actions of ginkgo made sense to me, and in many ways they still do. I liked both its antioxidant and blood flow activities, especially as it was believed that a vascular event might have contributed to my sudden hearing loss. My doctor was not overly optimistic, but he also did not object to my trying ginkgo. I started on the lower end of the dosage recommendation and tapered upward. Eventually, a pesky upset stomach, off-and-on headaches, and occasional dizziness made me think that this was not for me.

After about four months, I tapered off because I did not like the way I felt. I cannot say that it really made a difference in the tinnitus loudness or annoyance. Had I been able to tolerate higher doses for a much longer period of time, maybe the results would have been different. Ginkgo enthusiasts might question the lack of my success by wondering if the brand that I used met the necessary potency and standardization requirements. According to the label, it did contain the required 24 percent ginkgo flavone glycosides and 6 percent terpene lactones. However, as herbal products are not subject to FDA regulation, the manufacturer's word alone is our warranty. Potency and quality are two issues that plague the herbal and supplement industries in general.

Even though ginkgo is a natural product, it has possible side effects, drug interactions, and contraindications. Those who decide to try it should notify their physician and pharmacist, so that it can be added to their medication profile. Due to its effects on blood flow and blood clotting, ginkgo must be used cautiously in people with cardiovascular, bleeding, or blood-clotting issues. Ginkgo can reinforce the action of blood thinners. Before trying ginkgo, it is best to consult with the physician first. Also, if surgery is planned, it is important to check with the doctor on how long before the procedure ginkgo should be stopped and how soon afterward it can be resumed.

Chapter 28
Excessive Noise Sensitivity:
Recruitment and Hyperacusis

Tinnitus was not the only aggravating condition that followed my sudden hearing loss. Extreme noise sensitivity followed shortly. The conspiracy between recruitment and hyperacusis set me up for some tough times.

Three weeks after my initial hearing loss, I returned to the ENT clinic for repeat hearing tests and a visit with the specialist. It turned out to be a bittersweet day. As I mentioned earlier, my hearing had actually improved enough for a word recognition test to be added. I scored an amazing 28 percent, which showed that some healing had obviously taken place. Although the test results were encouraging, they did not explain why I had such extreme noise sensitivity. I could accept that in these early stages, the quality of my regained hearing left a lot to be desired, but why was everything so awfully loud? What I heard of the real world can only be described as a scary mess of mostly unhelpful cacophony. I wondered if I would have to live forever in this inferno. I wore out the TV mute button, as there were few sounds that did not make me cringe and want to run. Outside, I wore industrial-quality earplugs for personal safety reasons. Startled by a noise, I could have easily jumped into the street, only to get run over by the proverbial bus. The audiologist tried to reassure me that in my situation, this was not unusual. With any luck, things would settle down over time. She talked about a gradual, guarded improvement.

Dr. Leonard nodded his head as he reviewed the test tracings. He seemed satisfied yet surprised. He mentioned that he never thought that I would regain "this much hearing." I told him that the squiggles on the piece of paper belied reality and that not everything in my hearing world was well. I asked if some of my new challenges might be the result of my progress; I could hardly tolerate sound. The better right ear was even getting into the fray, as it felt that there was noise carry-over from the left to the right. Road noise drove me berserk. High frequencies had become my enemies. Shrieking children sent me running. The piercing sounds would hit my ear and scatter. Restaurants turned into painful halls of torture. I either heard little, or it was way too loud, blurred and without definition.

The doctor felt that I probably had two different things going on at once: possibly recruitment mixed with a touch of hyperacusis. I was not familiar with the concept of recruitment.

Recruitment

The fast loudness escalation—from little to boom—could be assigned to a phenomenon known as "recruitment. " It is often a result of cochlear hair cell damage or death. The more cell devastation there is, the worse the recruitment issue will be. As I had a pronounced decline in the upper frequencies, it would make sense that I had also quite a bit of recruitment going on in those ranges. According to the doctor, this was a very complicated process that even specialists had trouble sorting out.

Here is my pared-down, bare-bones version that helped me understand how recruitment works, at least in very general terms. Normally, cochlear cells are tuned to respond to specific frequency stimuli. When my cochlea was attacked, a good portion of the hearing cells took a beating, especially those in the upper-frequency ranges. Some were damaged, while others died. The cochlear cell carpet now showed areas of heavy wear and tear, as well as bald spots or dead zones. This meant that my brain got spotty and imperfect sound signals from the impaired frequency zones. Unsatisfied with such faulty input, the brain activated nature's backup plan for filling in the sound blanks. The backup plan was called "recruitment."

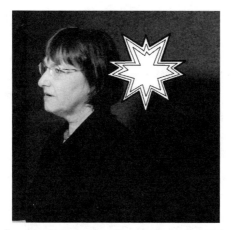

The author describes recruitment: when the sound goes from tolerable to BOOM!
The sound seems to burst inside the ear. *photo: R.Hammond*

In recruitment, functioning cells adjacent to those that are incapacitated are called upon, or *recruited,* to fill in for their neighbors. Now the recruits must fire on their own behalf as well as pick up the slack for surrounding non-responders. Depending on how serious the devastation is, they might be deputized to take on ever more assignments, thus doing two, three, or more jobs besides their own. The "stand-ins," however, also operate a lot outside of their tuned comfort zones. Suddenly, there is a whole lot of chiming going on, much of it not in tune. In practice, the cells' multi-tasking results in recruitment, a rapidly growing, confused sound response from the damaged frequency ranges.

Like most backup plans, the recruitment plan is not perfect, to say the least. The deputized cells do the best they can, but the quality of the resulting signal leaves a lot to be desired and can be quite unsettling to the patient. Recruited sound is not only loud, it is also unclear. Frequencies run together, which makes it difficult to separate words and to understand speech. Energetically loud mumbo-jumbo is what I mostly heard, at least in the beginning.

I wondered if this noise chaos might improve as more cells recuperated and took over their own duty. Obviously, that would depend on how many cells in the target frequencies were still capable of doing so. I was cautioned that any dead cells would not regenerate. They were dead. I might always have a recruitment issue in those pesky high frequencies. We would have to wait and see.

As my hearing improved ever so slowly, the almost intolerable din calmed down somewhat. Maybe my brain simply adjusted. Today, my headphones are no longer cemented to my ears. I actually go for walks without earplugs. My upper frequency losses are permanent, and some sound-scattering will remain a problem forever. Although newer hearing instruments might do a better job, a couple of audiologists have told me that I can blame recruitment, at least partially, for the fact that hearing aids are not very helpful to me. This is why I am grateful for every decibel and for every hertz that I regained on my own. As further improvement is no longer expected, it looks like this is as good as it gets.

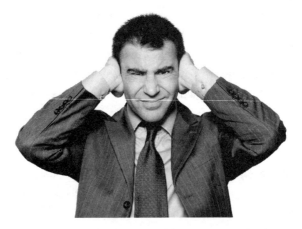

Hyperacusis: when the world seems way too loud.
photo: (c) Ostill www.fotosearch.com

Hyperacusis

Loosely translated the word "hyperacusis" means "super-loud hearing." I knew of hyperacusis as a possible side effect of certain medications, migraines, or head injuries. I was, however, unaware of its ties to hearing loss and tinnitus. That said, one does *not* need to have a hearing loss in order to have hyperacusis. Work done by audiologist Marsha Johnson highlights the complexities and challenges of this rather bothersome condition. Dr. Johnson describes two types of hyperacusis: cochlear hyperacusis and vestibular hyperacusis. The cochlear version has sound/hearing connections. The vestibular version has sound/balance connections.

Cochlear Hyperacusis or Hyperacusis

Cochlear hyperacusis, which is often simply referred to as "hyperacusis," is an exaggerated, abnormal sensitivity to everyday sounds. Everything is too loud. The sound of a passing car or of a coffeemaker chugging along could be excruciating to a person. The brain's internal volume control seems to have lost the low or medium settings. Sounds that are part of daily life and that others perceive as normal can cause distress to those with cochlear hyperacusis, from discomfort to pain or torture. Noises that come through as overly loud can precipitate serious emotional responses. Some people need medication to help them control the anxiety and stress that hyperacusis can cause. It is easy to see why people who suffer from this condition could become hermits, hiding from life. My case was by no means that serious, but it was unpleasant nevertheless.

The list of suspected causes for cochlear hyperacusis is extensive and varied. Loud-noise exposures and head injuries resulting in damage to the inner ear are always prime suspects. It could be a medication side effect or the result of exposure to certain toxins. Autoimmune disorders have been implicated. Derangement of the middle ear ossicle chain, subsequent to head trauma, could possibly lead to such sound over-amplification. Otosclerosis can cause people to become overly sound-sensitive. Sudden hearing loss due to viral damage of the eighth cranial nerve can also result in hyperacusis. People with TMJ or migraines tend to complain of sound intolerance for reasons not well understood. Autism also commonly involves excessive sound sensitivity. Another mystery is that a good portion of those who have tinnitus also have cochlear hyperacusis.

In the absence of a physical cause, scientists question whether hyperacusis might be due to a glitch in how the brain perceives and processes sounds. Maybe brain chemistry issues could contribute to the noise over-expression. Links to psychological or psychiatric conditions have also been sought. In short, there are currently still more questions than there are answers. In my case, the assumption was that hyperacusis could play a part in my sound intolerance. My ear had been through a lot of trauma and all the insults created a hyperacusis-friendly environment.

Specialists agree that people who are plagued by unusual sound sensitivity and whose lives are adversely affected by it should have a medical evaluation by an ear expert. There are no specific tests for hyperacusis, but our health history can provide the specialist with valuable information. The menu of tests that are ordered for evaluating a hyperacusis patient includes many of those that had been performed on me: a physical check, blood work, an ear inspection, a full set of hearing assessments, and an MRI of the head. A psychological evaluation can also be added.

After my doctor's visit, I discussed my hyperacusis issue with an audiologist who had some interesting insights. I confessed to having had a problem with high-pitched sounds all of my life. Ever since childhood, I reacted in a negative way to those types of noises. While hyperacusis was a definite possibility, the audiologist believed that my lifetime condition might well be *misophonia,* which means *a dislike of certain sounds.* We all have a bit of that—there are noises and pitches that just rub us the wrong way. Yet misophonia can become overwhelming under certain conditions. For me, it deepened the challenges of a situation that involved recruitment in my frequency "dislike-zone." By the time I added the effects of recruitment to those of hyperacusis and threw in a pinch of aggravated tinnitus, it was no wonder that I felt like living in a nerve-racking noise inferno. Physical issues compounded by emotional prejudices made for a challenging mix. The audiologist discussed some desensitization strategies with me, and I decided that, as my condition allowed, I would try to rein in my emotional bias and normalize my attitude toward my problem pitches. I would start softly and see where it would take me. I found out that old habits die hard.

Desensitize and Normalize

The same principles that apply to treating tinnitus also apply to cochlear hyperacusis. Those whose lives are seriously affected by the condition can find professional help at an audiology clinic that specializes in TRT (tinnitus retraining therapy). Besides tinnitus, TRT also addresses the issue of hyperacusis. Again, the goal is to train the brain to adapt, to become more tolerant to noise, and to normalize its responses. If people have both tinnitus and hyperacusis, hyperacusis is addressed first. However, a medical evaluation is still needed before one can proceed.

Although white noise might be helpful, *pink noise* is preferred for treating hyperacusis patients. "Pink noise" is mostly made up of frequencies that dominate daily life. It is not liberally spiked with high pitches the way white noise is. Wearable noise generators are sold by audiologists and commercial pink-noise CDs are also available. Even those who decide on home treatment, however, do well to talk to an

217

audiologist for guidance on available sound treatment options and the appropriate use of sound-producing devices. One does not want to make the situation worse inadvertently.

Beware of Overprotection

Sound sensitivity entices people to overprotect their ears, as I well know. The doctor had already warned me not to fall into that trap. There is a balance between suffering and overprotection, he said. The theory is that the more one locks out *all* noise, the less one will be able to tolerate *any* noise at all. I could see how this might be severely limiting from a social point of view and a sure set-up for anxiety and panic reactions. I heeded the advice. Except for situations like being in the noisy kitchen with several appliances running at once, or when using the vacuum cleaner or the hair dryer, I quit using earplugs or noise-reducing headphones around the house or when visiting family or friends. I replaced my industrial plugs with lighter ones that I still wear to the store or in the car on challenging days. I went for as long as I possibly could without ear protection in otherwise decibel-safe environments. I gradually improved, and at this point I feel almost normal again. I rarely wear ear plugs anymore—although I always carry them with me—and the headphones are getting a well-deserved rest, at least most of the time.

At this point, I am able to listen—still very cautiously—to music that incorporates flutes and violins. Compared to the ruckus that I lived in before, this is progress, something to build on. My reintroduction into the world of song—male artists only, sorry—began when my husband got me a couple of CDs with *Elvis* singing Christmas songs. Now that was serious medicine. Then again, the King has sung me through all of my life's crises, so why stop now?

Vestibular Hypercusis—When Sound Affects Balance

Vestibular hyperacusis is a most interesting yet unsettling

condition. Exposure to sound can bring about an upset in the balance system. Certain tones may trigger attacks in patients that render them unable to retain their posture or their balance, and they fall down as a result. There are also those who can be overcome by sudden episodes of vertigo or nausea in response to sound exposure. Confusion, extreme fatigue, and headaches have also been reported.

There is a lot that must still be learned about vestibular hyperacusis. From what is known so far, basically anything that damages the organs themselves or the nerve cells within the balance system could set off the condition. Head and neck trauma figure among the leading causes, but adverse reactions to certain chemicals or medications, and oxygen depletion due to heart and circulation issues are also suspected, as are possible autoimmune connections.

Descriptions of being thrown off-kilter or of being made ill by noises are sure to draw incredulous looks from anyone, unfamiliar with vestibular hyperacusis, which even applies to physicians. It is frustrating for patients to be told that their symptoms testify to a psychological event, when there might actually be a physical explanation for them.

It is important for people with symptoms of vestibular hyperacusis to seek out an expert in ear disorders for checking on possible causes. Conversely, a specialized hyperacusis clinic might shed some light on the issue. Because this is such an elusive condition, it makes sense to keep a diary. Information with as much detail as possible might put the doctor or audiologist on the right track. An accurate description of symptoms, when and how they started, and how long an episode lasts is a good beginning. It also helps to specify what type of noise triggers an event and what special places, if any, might be trouble spots. Blocking known offending noises by means of earplugs or headphones is a strategy that has reportedly been beneficial. It also helps to think of possible causes, such as a recent viral infection, surgery, head or neck issues, new medications or supplements, and so on.

So far there is no effective way to test for vestibular hyperacusis. For the patient, it is important not to give up. The hard part is to find a physician or audiologist who is familiar with the condition, who reads and interprets the symptoms correctly, who knows which tests might help to track a cause, and who can advise the client on strategies for getting relief and for preventing injuries due to falls.

PART FOUR

HEARING INSTRUMENT BASICS:
STYLES, TECHNOLOGY, SALES

Chapter 29
Authorized to Buy a Hearing Aid and My First Hearing Aid Class

About three months after my initial ear event, the audiograms showed that my hearing had reached a steady state. Short of a miracle, further positive changes were unlikely to happen. During a routine office visit, Dr. Leonard finally gave me the green light to try a hearing aid. I wondered why he was not more excited. I sure was. My hearing was going to be digitally remastered, and this was a big day for me. It was also the day that I found out that doctors are not that much into hearing aids. Dr. Leonard simply said that I could consider checking on a device. It might help or it might not.

I asked what type of hearing aid he thought would be most beneficial to me. The doctor did not have any specific suggestions; in fact, he would not be involved with the choosing, fitting, or programming of a device. He stated that recommending an appropriate instrument and programming the correct settings would be the job of a hearing specialist, such as an audiologist or hearing aid dispenser, and he wished me good luck in finding a "compatible" one. Dr. Leonard felt that I would be best served by a community-based hearing aid store. I would have to shop around. He did, however, recommend a consultation with a clinic audiologist for a hearing aid initiation lesson. At least I would get a basic understanding of how the audiogram and the choice of a hearing device interplayed. This was great advice, and I decided to follow through on the suggestion.

Ultimately, I received copies of my tests, together with a signed medical release for the hearing aid vendor. This statement certified that the causes for my hearing loss had been duly investigated by a medical specialist. It allowed me to venture out in search of hearing assistance. The doctor expressed hope that my bundle of papers might get the process started on the right track.

My suspicions were justified; this was the end of Dr. Leonard's involvement. I had expected to receive a written order with specific tuning instructions for the hearing aid expert—a prescription of sorts. But it did not work that way. With papers in hand, but otherwise defenseless and clueless, I was released into the "hearing aid jungle."

Suddenly, all the decisions were up to me. There was no safety net. I was on my own, but I was also most eager to explore what kind of assistance modern technology might offer. I had been told that depriving the injured ear of targeted, adjusted sound input might cause it to deteriorate further. The slogan of "use it or lose it" came to mind. There was no denying that the search for better hearing would take a lot of patience and plenty of professional expertise.

Although the doctor made sure that I would not delay getting help, it takes many people with hearing loss an average of seven years before they act on their symptoms. Even getting tested does not mean that they will invest in hearing aids or assistive devices. Meanwhile, the ears continue to weaken due to *auditory deprivation*.

As a newcomer to hearing loss and all of its side issues, I had a lot to learn. My dream was that I would get to hear better immediately. I had seen too many ads with smiling, satisfied customers. This could be me. I was sure that one of those miniaturized, digital, "intelligent" instruments would get my life back on track, right now.

My search for better hearing definitely had its ups and downs, and it still does. It turned out to be a rather pricey and often frustrating ride on the hope/disappointment/hope roller coaster. Of course, everybody's experience is different. The more uncomplicated the hearing loss, the easier it is to get help. I had been warned that I might run into some hiccups. And I did. I would find out that getting a hearing aid is not only a major purchase, it is also a journey that demands patience, cooperation, and commitment from both the patient and the instrument practitioner—the team for success.

My First Hearing Aid Class: Five College Credits in One Hour!

As advised by Dr. Leonard, my first venture took me to the audiology clinic affiliated with the doctor's office. I came away a bit more sober but with a lot more information and confidence. My initial hearing aid consult was not a sales pitch. Instead, it was an informal, low-pressure way for me to become familiar with instrument features, technical details, and technical expressions that tend to overwhelm the uninitiated. It also offered an opportunity for a one-on-one question-and-answer exchange with an unbiased professional.

Looking back, I am extremely grateful to my mentor, audiologist Denise. She was very professional, informative, and realistic. In the course of our discussions I learned a few important lessons.

No Cure for Hearing Loss

I learned that hearing aids do not cure hearing loss and that, even under the best of circumstances, my hearing would never again be the way it was. A sensorineural loss is irreversible. Hearing aids, no matter how pricey, do not restore normal hearing. They can help us make the most out of the hearing that we have left, but they are not a "fix." How effective these devices are depends on the type and extent of the hearing loss and on the expertise of the instrument practitioner.

I hasten to add, however, that thanks to advances in hearing aid technology, many patients report hearing clarity and increases in quality of life beyond their wildest dreams. They hear sounds like a bird chirping or their own footsteps that they had not heard for ages. These little gizmos can restore one's functioning in social and professional settings to a degree that was impossible just a short time back.

Amplification and Sensitivity Issues

Next, I learned that hearing aids are basically amplifiers that can be tuned to accommodate a variety of hearing shortcomings under different circumstances. Typically, milder, uncomplicated hearing losses are easiest to address, but even the newest and best of technologies have limits. The new digital instruments allow for the most flexibility. Although Denise felt that I could benefit from such a device, my combination of high frequency loss and noise-sensitivity issues gave her cause for concern. She mentioned that getting enough meaningful amplification in the higher ranges was often difficult to achieve and could pose a challenge in noise-sensitive clients. Because of the recruitment and hyperacusis, any amplification might very well make things worse, especially the tinnitus.

Although some people's tinnitus can be helped by a hearing aid, it is always hard to predict the outcome. Denise expressed hope that my situation would be manageable, as audiologists deal with these challenges all the time. I was cautioned, however, to get ready for a series of trips to the place of sale, as multiple adjustments could be expected. It suddenly dawned on me that getting a hearing aid was a trifle more involved than I had thought.

Real-ear Measures

One comment that I found interesting was that not all sound that is processed by the instrument might reach the eardrum. Therefore, the hearing aid specialist should perform real-ear measures. After the instrument is set, a tiny probe is introduced into the ear canal. It will measure the actual sound outputs at the receiver, or loudspeaker, level. Often, there is conflict between what the computer programs show and what is actually delivered to the eardrum. If the probe's findings do not match the computer information, there could be an electronic problem somewhere along the path.

In my many visits with audiologists and hearing instrument dispensers, no one ever used such a probe. I asked about this various times, but I never received a satisfactory answer as to how and if real-ear measures had been performed. Some fitters seem to incorporate them routinely into the process, while others do not. Yet it would make sense that such measures might speed up the adjustment process and save on trips to the clinic.

Importance of Lifestyle

Next, the audiologist interviewed me about my lifestyle. She asked under what circumstances a hearing aid would be of most help to me—at work, socializing, or at home. She inquired about the types of sports or activities that I enjoyed. She was also interested whether I cared if the instrument was visible on the outside. Lifestyle and personal preferences all play important parts in the choice of a hearing aid.

The Occlusion effect, Venting, and Acoustic Feedback

I asked Denise what might be causing an annoying clunking noise whenever I walked while wearing an earplug in my left ear. Every time I put my foot down—clunk, clunk. I could not imagine having a hearing device stuck in my ear canal. The clunking was due to what is known as the *occlusion effect*. Because of the earplug blockage, low-frequency sound waves became trapped and bounced back and forth between the earplug and the eardrum. Without a way to escape to the outside, these waves were amplified by bone conduction, which accounted for them being rather loud. I could consider loosening the earplug fit, which would allow for more normalized sound flow. Protecting the ears was good, but I also needed to use common sense.

Yet I still wondered how the clunking would affect hearing aid use. Occlusion does become an issue with hearing instruments that either fit tightly into the ear canal or involve the use of tight earmolds. Such blockages trap already amplified sounds that are further magnified through bone conduction. People often report that their head feels like an echo chamber and that their own voice sounds weird, dull, and often excessively loud.

227

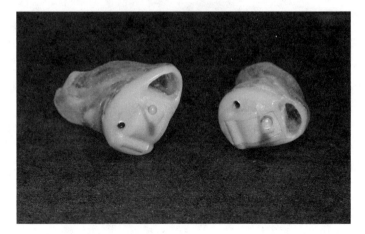

A hearing aid vent can prevent sound from being trapped inside the ear canal.
Trapped sound can produce a thumping when walking. *photo: R.Hammond*

Venting is a technique for dealing with occlusion caused by hearing devices. The problem due to amplified, bouncing sound waves can be alleviated by simply making a small hole, or vent, into the aid's shell or earmold. The idea is to let some of the low-frequency waves escape gently to the outside. However, the size of the vent puts limits on this technique. The larger the opening, the more sound leaks from the ear canal to the outside, which makes the hearing device inefficient. For people who need all the amplification they can get across all frequencies, letting sound "drain" out through venting has its definite limits. What's more, vented, already amplified sound waves contribute to *acoustic feedback*. They are picked up once more by the hearing aid's microphone and are put through yet another round of amplification. This becomes a vicious cycle that leads eventually to embarrassing *acoustic feedback* squeals. While venting can solve some issues, it can also easily lead to others.

A poorly fitted hearing aid can also contribute to acoustic feedback. Already amplified sounds that leak to the outside from around the instrument are re-fed through the microphone and re-amplified. Ear wax plugs that bounce back sound waves from the hearing aid can

228

also help produce the screams, as can instruments that are turned up way too loud.

Feedback is a particular problem for people with a severe hearing loss who need serious amplification. Once the whistling starts, the natural reflex is to turn the volume down. This is also how hearing aid specialists might make adjustments in order to tweak the squeak, especially in older style instruments. But then the patient loses needed amplification and hears less. Fortunately, there are newer options.

Feedback Cancellation

Denise mentioned that I would not have a problem with occlusion because my hearing loss allowed for a vented or open-fit hearing aid. She added that by letting air circulate, such instruments provide greater comfort as they cut down on ear humidity, a common cause of ear itchiness due to closed, tightly fitting devices. Also, feedback should not be a concern because, in this digital age, hearing aids are routinely equipped with special circuitry that cancels acoustic feedback. This makes instruments more efficient because the volume can be turned up without running instantly into whistling issues. As our acoustic environments change continuously, tiny micro-analysts scan the hearing aid output fast and furiously for sound bits that could cause the notorious squeak. As all of this work has to be done at a rapid pace in the here-and-now, a hearing aid user may occasionally perceive some slight sound distortion. These systems are not foolproof and occasionally make a wrong decision in their efforts to tame and to eliminate annoying squeals.

Importance of Communication

The audiologist had another very important message for me: communicate! It is our job to inform the hearing specialist how an instrument feels or sounds to us. If we are bothered by problems regarding fit, sound quality, or feedback, we must speak up. If we have style preferences, we should mention them, and the specialists will try their best to accommodate us. Only the clients can provide the relevant information and input that help the expert choose a suitable device and program it to meet our needs. I was told that the instrument specialist and I would become a team as we endeavored to get the best possible results.

Give It a Chance

I was urged to give my hearing aid a chance to prove itself. In general, the first setting is not the best one or the final one. Denise felt that my chances for making multiple trips to the vendor were exceptional. She suggested that I might include the distance to the audiology clinic among my search criteria. I also had to be aware, she said, that it would take a while to get used to the new "way of hearing," and that every new setting would require a new "training period." The brain had to adapt. Lastly, Denise admonished me not to put my device in a drawer and forget it. I was to welcome it into my life and befriend it.

Take Good Care of It

Finally, the point was made that cautious handling and good care prolong the life of the device. It is better to get a larger aid than one that is too small and tricky to manipulate. Crashes to the floor can wreck the circuitry, and repairs are expensive. As a hearing aid is a pricey investment, Denise felt that it would be in my favor to extend its usefulness by keeping it clean and dry. Because wax and moisture are the two enemies of any hearing aid, the instrument must be stored according to the manufacturer's instructions and not just be tossed onto the kitchen counter.

Prices and Paperwork

Denise cautioned me that prices among hearing aids varied greatly.

Although people are often led into buying too much technology, more might not necessarily be better. I was told to ask the specialist for details on the features of a recommended device, inquire how and why they might help me, and express my financial concerns. Most of all, I should read the sales contract very carefully and make sure that I understood the trial period, service contract, warranty, refund policies and payment agreements. I asked about shopping for better prices at a sales event. My mentor, however, did not believe that these were good starting points for beginners because the focus was understandably more on sales than on patient education.

***

After this lengthy introduction to hearing loss and hearing aids, I was exhausted. As it turned out, an hour was not enough time, but I had learned a lot, although not all of it necessarily encouraging. The audiologist advised me to think about our conversation and to visit some regular hearing aid shops. This would help me get an idea of the different types of devices, prices, and manufacturers. I would also get a feeling for the various specialists' approaches to my challenges. I came away from our session with plenty of valuable food for thought.

I was glad to go home and spend some time digesting all of these convoluted circuitry noodles and computer chips. There were so many options out there. It seemed to me that I needed an experienced specialist more than I needed extra microprocessors. And dollar signs had me reeling. Certainly, the technology was out there but I needed to make a financial analysis and decide how much of the family discretionary income I wanted to stick into my ear.

Nowadays, one can buy price-reduced hearing aids online—often without much of a hearing test—that people can adjust themselves. Special apps for such self-tuning efforts are reported to become available in the not-so-distant future. Considering all my ear challenges and technology shortcomings, I have not tried this approach. So far, I still believe in professional hearing tests and rely on the help of an audiologist. My lack of know-how makes me worry that I might inadvertently damage my hearing further. However, this does not mean that I will not give it a try in the future.

Chapter 30
Hearing Aid Types and Styles

Hearing devices have been around for some time. When I was a child, I went with my family to visit the birthplace of Ludwig van Beethoven in Bonn, Germany. Beethoven, of course, was a genius of a composer who went deaf later on in his life and who was also plagued by tinnitus. I will never forget being totally befuddled by the display of his "hearing trumpet" collection. As Beethoven held the tapered instrument neck to his ear, people would speak loudly into the round, open end of the trumpet. The sound would concentrate as it traveled down the thinning shaft into the ear canal. I cannot even imagine the torture that this must have been. Any hearing cells that still had some life in them were sure to be silenced by this "scream louder" strategy.

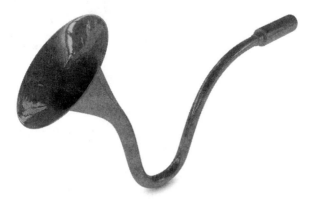

The ear trumpet was used before electronic hearing aids.
photo: (c) pixelfabrik www.fotosearch.com

Overall, the ear trumpet was a crude way of increasing sound pressure or loudness. For many people with hearing loss, however, louder is not necessarily better. It certainly isn't for me. Yet these very basic mechanical devices were considered to be an improvement over what there was before—nothing. Yelling at the afflicted or totally ignoring and excluding them from society were common practice. All things considered, I feel fortunate to live in a time of medical and technological enlightenment.

As I stared at the exhibit in the glass case, little did I know that so many years later I would go hunting for a more upscale hearing trumpet of my own.

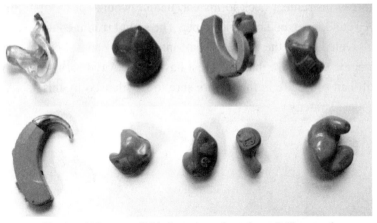

Hearing Aids are available in many styles. *photo: R.Hammond*

The hearing aids that we commonly see in use are *air conduction* devices, which are particularly well suited for losses that are sensorineural in nature. Sound information flows freely through the ear from the pinna to the cochlea. Air conduction instruments, however, often do not work the best for people with a conductive hearing loss. Depending on the case, those patients might benefit from a *bone conduction instrument.*

As technology races ahead, the basic styles for modern-day hearing instruments have not changed that much, even though the trend is to aim for invisibility, comfort, clarity, and versatility. Thanks to new case materials and circuitry, instruments have become smaller and faster in their sound-processing capabilities. They have also moved beyond their main jobs of amplifying and modulating sound and now have electronic applications, or "apps." They can have wireless features, be cell phone- and Bluetooth-compatible, FM-integrated, and so on. Some models are supplied with their own control devices that let them communicate directly with the TV. Ultimately, the hearing aid specialist helps us determine which device will serve us best. The following diagrams show the approximate position or location of the various styles of instruments.

Behind-The-Ear (BTE) instruments

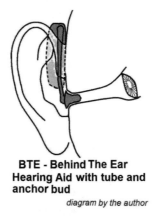

**BTE - Behind The Ear
Hearing Aid with tube and
anchor bud**
diagram by the author

The *traditional* behind-the-ear (BTE) style instrument is widely used and can accommodate any type of hearing loss, from mild to profound. These are rather sturdy, versatile, and powerful devices. They "hook" onto the top of the ear by means of a curved plastic extension to which plastic tubing with an anchor bud are attached. The instrumentation is contained in a small case that is worn behind the ear. The shell has space available for added electronic features, should they be needed. BTE instruments are supplied with manual controls for volume adjustments or for switching between listening programs.

Sound penetrates the ear through the plastic tube, which is secured in the ear canal by the anchor bud. As these instruments are used to assist with more severe degrees of hearing loss, the tube runs traditionally through a custom-made earmold. This means that the hearing aid specialist must take ear impressions to assure that the mold has the fit necessary for sealing off the ear canal. Common earmold issues relate to comfort and occlusion.

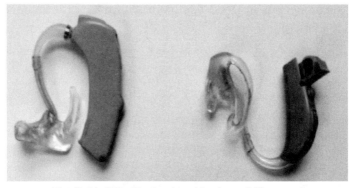

Two Behind The Ear hearing aids *photo: R.Hammond*

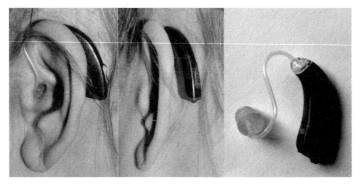

Three views of a Behind the Ear Hearing Aid. *photo: R.Hammond*

BTEs can be equipped with proprietary, manufacturer-specific plug-in ports that let the user connect directly with other external sources—CD or MP3 player, phone, computer, speaker microphone, or TV—by means of special cables and adapters known as "boots" or "shoes." This means that the device has a *direct audio input (DAI)*. FM adapters (boots) are also available for wireless connections. It is worthwhile to check on the DAI feature; many people do not know that their instrument is thus enabled. The connection points are visible on the bottom of the instrument shell. Usually, the DAI mode switches the hearing aid's microphone off. This eliminates background and interference noises, which makes for a clearer signal. Yet there are also options that allow for the hearing instrument's microphone to stay on, in case clients want to also stay aware of what is going on around them.

I know of students who use the wireless FM DAI adapter in noisy classrooms, where the teacher's voice is barely audible to them. The teacher wears a clip-on microphone that connects to a transmitter pack. The microphone signal is transmitted to FM boots that have been slipped onto the bottom of the student's BTE hearing aids. The teacher can move about the room and the student hears, wirelessly, without the continued strain of keeping track of the teacher, attempting to read lips (speech read), and interpret body language. What a difference this can make in the quality of a child's education.

The *mini* or *thin-tube BTE* is a smaller, lighter version of the traditional BTE. It does not have an "ear hook." The amplified sound is conducted into the ear by means of a plastic tube that is thinner and less obtrusive than the tube of the sturdier model. Depending on the type and severity of the hearing loss, the mini BTE can be equipped with an earmold, or the ear canal can be left open, which is known as "open-fit."

For the open-fit version, the tube is anchored in the ear canal by means of a vented tip or bud, located at the end of the tube. As the ear canal is left open, occlusion is eliminated and the ear remains drier, which is a plus for clients with itchy ears or for those who are prone to infections. My first instrument was a thin-tube, open-fit device. I liked it, but I had trouble with the anchor fixture that seemed to dislocate easily, especially as the plastic tube warmed to body temperature. Trying different bud sizes did not seem to make much difference, as the aid kept falling off.

An extremely popular open-fit BTE is the *Receiver-in-the-Canal (RIC)* model. The big change is that the loudspeaker, or receiver, has been removed from the main case. It is embedded in a protective pad at the end of a thin, shielded transmission *wire*—not a tube—that penetrates into the ear canal. The receiver is further held in position by means of a soft, vented tip. This configuration allows for concentrated sound to reach the eardrum. The signal is stronger and clearer than that of the regular open-fit BTE, where sound dissipates to some degree as it travels through a tube to the eardrum. For people with a more severe hearing loss, earmolds can be fitted which will prevent sound leakage and allow for an extra power boost.

Separating the microphone from the receiver has virtually eliminated feedback. It also has further miniaturized the hearing aid. By now, some models are as big as large almonds and fit more over the ear than behind the ear. As durability has been sacrificed to some extent for unobtrusiveness, patients must learn how to insert and remove these instruments cautiously. It is important not to force or pull the wires. Wires snap easily and may not be covered by the warranty.

As the receiver is no longer protected inside the hearing aid and is exposed to the humidity in the ear, proper dry storage when not in use is important in order to prolong its life-span. Replacing the receiver is easy enough to do but such repairs can be costly.

In-The-Ear (ITE) Devices

To fashion in-the-ear devices with a snug but comfortable fit, the hearing aid specialist must take ear impressions. Unless they are vented, occlusion can be an issue with these devices; yet venting may lead to feedback problems. For in-the-ear hearing aids, the circuitry is located in a shell that rests in the outer portion of the ear, known as the ear bowl, or concha.

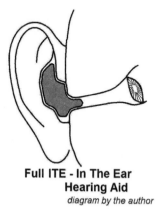

**Full ITE - In The Ear
Hearing Aid**
diagram by the author

There are two ITE versions: the *full-size* device fills the entire ear bowl, while the *half-shell* fills only the lower half of the ear bowl. To make them less obvious, the color of the shell matches the wearer's skin tone as closely as possible. Due to their size, ITEs are well suited for clients with limited finger dexterity. They are routinely equipped with manual control buttons.

Ear-Canal Instruments

Designing hearing instruments that fit somewhere inside the ear canal calls for the specialist to take ear canal impressions. As these devices hide deeper and deeper within the canal, they are programmed to work automatically on their own with a minimum, if any, intervention from the wearer. Manual adjustments are no longer feasible for some styles, yet, if necessary, remote control devices can be used for this purpose.

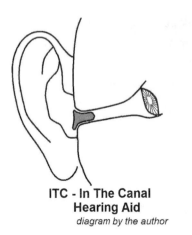

ITC - In The Canal Hearing Aid
diagram by the author

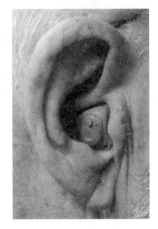

An In The Canal hearing aid fits just inside the ear canal *photo: R.Hammond*

In-the-canal (ITC) hearing aids fit in the outermost part of the ear canal. They are smaller and a lot less visible than ITEs. Although manual control features are still used for these aids, they are a lot trickier to handle.

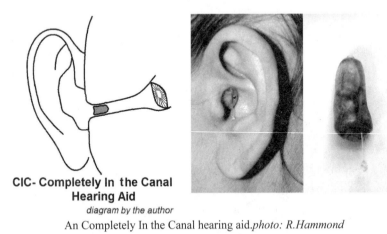

CIC- Completely In the Canal Hearing Aid
diagram by the author
An Completely In the Canal hearing aid.*photo: R.Hammond*

Completely-in-the-canal (CIC) instruments are sought after because they are quite small and hardly visible. People with narrow or somewhat contorted ear canals are hard to fit. If these instruments are not seated just right, they easily become uncomfortable. The mere action of talking or chewing can dislocate the device. Patients who are prone to frequent ear infections or who produce lots of earwax are not considered good CIC candidates. Unless they are vented, occlusion becomes a problem. Handling the instrument and changing tiny batteries can be a challenge. After trying various hearing aid designs, I ended up with a vented CIC. The first thing that broke on it was the fragile plastic ring that held the minuscule battery.

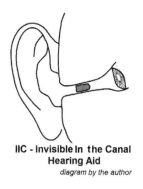

**IIC - Invisible In the Canal
Hearing Aid**
diagram by the author

The *invisible-in-the canal (IIC)* model is the micro-version of the CIC. These devices are quite slender and completely invisible. Inserted and changed by specially trained vendors, they snuggle farther into the ear canal and rest closer to the eardrum than the conventional CIC. It is important to inquire if showering or swimming with the instrument in place is allowed. The patient turns the device on and off or adjusts the volume by means of a remote control device. Depending on usage, batteries can last for months.

Chapter 31
Hearing Instrument Technology

Since Beethoven's time, hearing technology has advanced by leaps and bounds. Yet no matter how we twist and turn, in the end, hearing aids are based on the principles of sound amplification. Depending on the complexity of the technology, air conduction devices are of two basic electronic types: analog or digital.

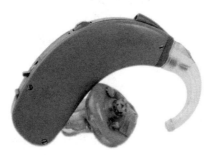

Although analog hearing aids do not look much different from the outside, their sound processing is less sophisticated than digital hearing aids. *photo: (c) Julenochek www.fotosearch.com*

Analog Hearing Aids

The sound waves of the world around us are without any refinement, ever-changing, blended, and continuous—they are in analog mode. Our ears pick up these sound waves and eventually convert them into electrical signals that are fed to the brain. We hear in analog mode, and so our ears are actually analog hearing organs. As our hearing decreases, incoming sound needs an added loudness boost by means of an amplifier. Enter the pioneers of the more modern-day hearing aid world—the analog hearing aids.

A *conventional* analog hearing device is also referred to as an "analog adjustable." It amplifies sound in a *linear* fashion, which means that all frequencies are made louder by the same amount. The amplification is the same across the board, whether it is speech, music, or background noise. Those who do the best with these devices are clients who have a relatively flat loss throughout the speech spectrum.

Obviously, if a loss is concentrated in a particular frequency range, like high or low frequencies, or if it changes across the different pitches, *everything* becoming louder is not a favorable outcome. The general increase in sound level becomes hard to tolerate. Although these instruments are sturdy, affordable, and have long battery life, it can be a challenge to find a comfortable loudness level for a given situation. People often report that the volume is either too low or too high and that they have to continuously adjust the instrument—simply because the analog hearing aid does not accommodate their hearing loss pattern.

A conventional analog aid is a battery-powered mini-loudspeaker system complete with microphone and sound amplifier. The microphone captures the sound from the environment and turns it into an electrical current, or signal. That signal travels to the amplifier, which increases or reinforces it. Next, the signal is relayed to the receiver, or loudspeaker, which reconverts the now boosted electrical signal back into sound—louder sound—that is then transmitted into the ear canal.

The manufacturing lab receives instructions for specific settings from the hearing expert, based on the client's audiogram. The basic electrical components are then rigged into the instrument shell. The patient can dial up or down on the volume or turn the hearing aid on or off by means of buttons or wheels located on the shell. The specialist is able to make limited corrections manually in the office. For more advanced changes or for repairs, the device must be returned to the factory. A special device called a telecoil (T-coil) facilitates phone conversations and is commonly installed in the hearing aid.

A modernized version is the *programmable analog.* Although it is more expensive, it offers a lot more flexibility than the conventional aid. It contains a basic microchip and already has limited digital capability. The specialist is able to change or adjust the settings in the office. By means of a computer, these instruments can be programmed for different listening situations, in accordance with the hearing test parameters and patient preferences. The user switches between the various programs, either manually by pressing a button on the device or by using a remote control.

Before my father lost his hearing aid, he kept "switching wavelengths" on his programmable analog device. Dad was a radio journalist, and his hearing specialist had explained the instrument's program features to him in terms that he could understand. When he came into the house, he reset his "hearing apparatus," as he called it, from the "outside" to the "inside" wavelength, or program. He also had a "conference" setting. I asked once what difference the various "wavelengths" made, and he replied that the switch changed the general hearing ambiance.

Analog technology is gradually being phased out as the new generations of digital devices flood the marketplace. This upsets those who love their analog instruments and who refuse to part with them. Yet there are also longtime users who could not wait to get rid of the analog "hearing-aid dinosaurs" and fully embrace digital technology. It all depends on our personality, type of hearing loss, what we are used to, to what we can best relate, and, ultimately, what we can afford.

Although analogs have been pushed aside by the new kids on the block—the digitals—some companies still make these instruments. For those who are interested in analog hearing aids, a conversation with the hearing specialist might be in order.

Digital Hearing Aids
Just like cars, digital hearing devices range from "stripped down"

to "fully loaded." There are four major, broadly defined categories: entry level, basic or economy, advanced, and premium. There are actual "digital grades" and not every one of these instruments is a deluxe model by definition.

The word "digital" has dealt a serious blow to our expectation management skills. The expression has almost become synonymous with sure-thing magic. But that is not necessarily so. Although the chances for getting hearing help are greatly increased with a digital aid, not all people benefit to their satisfaction from these devices. This said, digital hearing assistance is truly impressive, continues to improve, and has helped where other aids failed. In order to take full advantage of the advanced features of these instruments, however, practitioner experience and expertise are a must. Yet in the end, even the latest top-notch technology, no matter how expensive, can never match the natural hearing that we once had.

Digital aids are not as sturdy as their analog predecessors. They need gentler handling and more maintenance. Ever-decreasing sizes make them harder to manipulate. They are easy to drop. Plenty of finicky circuitry also contributes to their fragility, which calls for proper storage and regular cleaning care. With continuous use, they also burn through the batteries at a pretty fast pace. However, repair and battery expenses are often considered minor nuisances by those who have been helped beyond their expectations by these instruments.

The flexibility and adaptability of digital instruments are almost proverbial, but technology changes at lightning speed. We are told that nowadays hearing aids can tell the difference between speech and miscellaneous noise. They can be designed to interact wirelessly with *manufacturer-specific* electronics, such as computers, smartphones, watch-size computer devices and MP3 players. It is possible to "stream" information from such equipment directly to the hearing aids—a matched communication and information set. There seems to be no end to the tricks that these gadgets can be taught.

Microphones, as small as specks of black pepper, contribute a great deal to a hearing aid's listening quality. The standard omni-directional microphone picks up sounds from everywhere. This works fine for quieter locations, but it makes communication in noisy environments difficult. Nowadays, the hearing specialist can chose an instrument style that accommodates directional-microphone technology. A directional microphone amplifies the sound that is in front of us more than the sound that is in back of us, which produces a clearer speech signal in loud settings. To provide listening flexibility, hearing aids can be equipped with both omni-directional and directional microphones. Our lifestyle and listening requirements determine which microphone features we need most.

The Secret of Their Success: Sound Digitizing

Most hearing losses are not equal over all of the different frequencies that keep bombarding our ears. Some people have problems with the lower pitches. I have a rather steep loss in the upper frequencies. Others have sound voids in the mid-ranges. Every hearing loss is different, and we all need sound boosting and refining in different frequency areas. Digital or mathematical sound processing offers the best chance for getting a targeted, quality result.

A digital hearing aid is still an amplifier—but one with finesse. The basic components are the microphone, receiver, and battery. In addition, these devices are outfitted with all sorts of over-the-top microcircuitry, as well as high-tech, specialized, "intelligent", proprietary computer chips. The *digital signal processor* is considered the heart of the operation, and its preset parameters account for many of the differences between the hearing aids on the market.

A digital instrument breaks the incoming sound down into number strings, made of 0s and 1s. That process is called "digitizing." It provides the device with information on both pitch (frequency) and loudness. After the sound is decoded, the manufacturer-specific processor can begin its signal analysis and get busy with its sound-sculpting work. It gets its instructions from the hearing specialist, who is familiar with the features of the device.

Assisted by some highly complicated computer software, the expert can address the specifics of our hearing loss with a precision that analog technology does not allow. In a way, the practitioner selectively launders, amplifies, and manages our sound environment to fit our needs. Digitally polished sound is cleaner, crisper, and free of interference and distortion. Ultimately, the custom-manipulated signal is reconverted into analog mode by the receiver before it is fed back to the ear.

Hearing practitioners have become almost like "plastic surgeons of sound." They trim a bit here, augment a tad there. They compress, filter, and boost in order to make the miniature sound studios in or behind our ears work in our favor. In their instructions, manufacturers include complicated details about gain and compression options, bands and channels. But what does that mean to the client? During my first forays into the hearing aid world, I was clueless. The sound columns that appeared on the computer screen looked like a 3-D skyline of Manhattan. The touch of a wrong button could lead to quite a jam-up within my ear.

Digital micro-circuitry can become phenomenally complicated phenomenally fast. I had no idea what anybody was talking about and felt that I needed at least some understanding of the common catch-phrases that often spice up ads or obscure consults with hearing aid specialists—even though proprietary definitions, trade secrets, and manufacturer whims tend to confuse the picture.

Sound Makeover: Gain, Compression, Channels, Bands

In audiology, an increase in volume measured in decibels (dB) is called "gain." "Compression" is a method for preventing painful or annoying sounds from becoming too loud. Compression keeps the volume of such noises at acceptable preset levels.

The main advantage of digital hearing aids is that they provide a great deal of flexibility for remodeling signals to fit a given hearing loss. This is done by sectioning the frequency spectrum off into *bands* and *channels*. This tactic allows for highly specific sound manipulation. The expert can target individual frequencies without affecting others, which is an enormous advantage over older technology. In theory, the more sections there are, the more flexibility the audio specialist has for fine-tuning the settings.

Although different manufacturers might use bands and channels for different sound refining purposes, in extremely general terms, bands are for adjusting the gain of specific frequencies. Channels are programmed with compression characteristics. However, channels can also be assigned other noise-reduction and sound-management tasks. Obviously, manufacturers have their own specific ways for slicing the frequency pie.

There is no obvious standardization on how to subdivide the frequencies. Band and channel configurations depend on the *manufacturer's proprietary designs* for addressing different hearing loss areas. There is no magic number for how many bands and/or channels a device needs in order to be helpful. For example, two instruments with exactly the same band/channel numbers might behave totally differently because of the different organization or bundling of the frequencies. Although impressive for the consumer, higher numbers do not guarantee better sound quality in our individual case, but they do add to the cost. The secret for success lies mostly in *the way* the frequencies are lumped together and assigned their places within specific bands and channels. As clients, we want to know which instrument has the ideal band/channel frequency configurations that serve our hearing loss most effectively at an affordable price. In my case, tuning sections in the lower frequency ranges will sit idle. I don't need them, so why pay for them?

Generally speaking, people with a complex loss that affects a variety of frequencies require more bands and channels for optimum results than those who have a loss that affects only a specific area. As we do not want to pay for anymore technology than what we need, it is important to have a "band/channel" discussion with the instrument vendor.

Digital Memories or Programs

Just like the programmable analogs, digital technology also offers instruments with different "listening programs." The programs are often referred to as "memories." Each memory is mapped for a specific noise environment. One memory might store settings for our quiet home environment. Another one might be set for the frenetic workplace. Yet another could be tuned to adapt to noisy venues, such as restaurants or holiday parties.

The multiple-program feature can be a plus for those who have busy lives and must move quickly from one noise situation to another. However, it is quite important that the settings are clear and comfortable. It takes a bit of doing. The user can flip between the memories, either manually or by using a remote control. Some units also allow for limited adjustment control by letting the client modify the loudness within a program. If it is not possible for a patient to change the program manually, there are instruments that "sense" the environment that the person is in and switch automatically to the correct memory.

Bone-Conduction Hearing Aids

As I related earlier, during my very first hearing tests on the morning after I had suffered a sudden, left hearing loss, the audiologist attached a vibrator-type contraption to the back of my injured ear. It was held in place by means of a tight metal headband. My bone conduction hearing was being evaluated.

Unlike air conduction, bone conduction bypasses the outer ear and middle ear structures. Bone conduction hearing assistance applies to those patients who have a "conductive" hearing loss, which means that conventional air transmission of sound is hampered or interrupted due to issues of the outer and/or middle ear areas. Chronic infections, canal malformations or blockages, scarring caused by infections or surgery, cholesteatomas, and otosclerosis are some of the conditions that contribute to such a loss. Depending on the cause or seriousness of the case, patients with a conductive loss often find air conduction instruments to be less than effective. Bone conduction hearing aids might be able to help.

Bone conduction aids are battery-driven. These instruments do not have a receiver (loudspeaker). Sound waves captured by a microphone are transformed into an electrical signal, which is processed to fit the patients hearing needs. The adjusted signal is relayed to an oscillator that is applied to the bone behind the ear. The oscillator translates the electrical signal into vibrations. The vibrations travel through the skin and are picked up by the bones of the skull and jaw, which conduct them to the cochlea of the inner ear. In return, the cochlea converts the vibrations back into electrical signals that travel to the brain by means of the cochlear nerve.

One of the drawbacks of these instruments is that the *oscillator* (vibrator) must be applied firmly to the bone for the device to work. This is achieved by means of rather tight-fitting headbands that are often considered bulky and uncomfortable. People may complain of headaches and skin irritations due to the continuous pressure that is needed to maintain snug contact between the bone and the oscillator. Also, as vibrations travel through skin and tissue barriers, definition is invariably lost, which can lead to sound distortion and dulling. Early instruments looked much like the devices used during hearing tests. One method of making these aids less obtrusive was to build the circuitry and vibrator into spring-loaded bows of eyeglasses. Using eyeglasses as support for bone conduction equipment is still done today.

Bone conduction hearing aids, even though helpful and necessary, often failed to bring forth waves of excitement among users because of their relative complexity. However, like anything else in today's digital age, these devices also have undergone massive design and miniaturization makeovers. A compact unit that simplifies the bone conduction option houses the battery, microphone, digital sound-processing circuitry, T-coil, and vibrator, all in one. This eliminates the need for signal-transmission wires or cables. Such a unit can be worn on a headband, which applies especially to children or, as we shall see, it can vibrate the skull bones via implanted parts. Although still snug, nowadays headbands are made of more flexible materials that greatly ease the wearer's discomfort. Vibrations still travel through tissue barriers in the head-worn models, but the sound quality is said to be greatly improved when compared to the results of the vibrator pads of yesteryear.

***

Hearing Aid Battery Disposal: Keeping Nature Pristine

Hearing aids run on batteries. Although they are very small, such batteries should not be tossed into the general garbage. Like all batteries, they contain materials that are toxic to the environment. If they are buried in landfills, heavy metals leach into the soil and groundwater. If they are burned in incinerators, harmful compounds are released into the air that we breathe. Even though some companies now make "green" hearing aid batteries, we should err on the side of safety and dispose of them properly.

Spent or expired hearing aid batteries belong into a hazardous waste disposal container for drop-off or pick-up during special collection events, often organized by cities and counties. Those who do not have access to hazardous waste recycling opportunities might call on friends or family members to pass the "battery bag" along to the correct authorities for proper disposal.

Chapter 32
Buying a Hearing Aid:
Practitioners and Regulations

The purchase of a hearing aid is largely based on the trust that exists between the client and the vendor. Hearing instruments are complicated, highly technical devices that are also quite pricey. Yet the correct type and amount of hearing assistance can make a phenomenal difference in our lives. We owe it to ourselves to know the difference between the various professionals who counsel us and sell us improved quality of life in the form of better hearing. It is also important to appreciate that there are agencies that regulate and oversee the hearing aid business in an effort to protect us, the consumers.

Audiologists and Hearing Instrument Dispensers

People tend to refer to anyone who tests hearing or fits an instrument as an "audiologist." Although this might often be true, other hearing practitioners, called "hearing instrument dispensers" (HIDs), also serve clients with hearing loss. I found it helpful to familiarize myself with a few details regarding the qualifications and scope of practice of those who tend to us as we step into the hearing aid store, here in the U.S.

Audiologists are health care professionals trained to detect, diagnose, and manage problems related to hearing and balance. They have the highest level of education in their field, which gives them great flexibility in their professional choices. They take a standardized national test upon graduation from an accredited college or university and complete a required number of supervised clinical hours. Audiologists have at least a master's degree. As of 2007, those who want to qualify for the additional but voluntary board certification by the American Board of Audiology (ABA) must earn a doctorate degree in audiology (AuD). Some states have followed the ABA lead and now require an AuD for in-state practice licensing.

The American Speech-Language-Hearing Association (ASHA) also certifies audiologists with a Certificate of Clinical Competence in Audiology (CCC-A). As of January 1, 2012, applicants for the voluntary ASHA certification will also need a doctorate degree in audiology in order to qualify for certification. Many states require that audiologists also pass an additional hearing-aid dispensing test if they want to work in that area of practice.

Some audiologists enjoy working with patients, testing hearing, performing *diagnostic* assessments, and fitting and setting instruments. Others direct their attention to specialized fields of practice, research, education, and industry, or they may run their own hearing clinic. Tinnitus and hyperacusis clinics are generally headed by audiologists. In addition, audiologists work with implant teams and care for patients with implanted devices such as cochlear implants, middle ear implants, and bone-anchored hearing aids.

Hearing instrument dispensers (HIDs) are also authorized to practice by the state. Although practical and educational requirements vary greatly from state to state, a college degree is generally not required for entering the dispensing field. Typically, HID applicants get a state-prescribed amount of training in hearing aid stores or audiology clinics and take a written and practical exam to become state certified. Some states may administer their own certification tests, while others require that candidates pass a competency assessment offered by groups, such as the International Hearing Society (IHS). Qualified, already state licensed dispensers can become board certified by the National Board for Certification in Hearing Instrument Sciences (NBC-HIS). Upon passing the required exam administered by this board, dispensers can use the title of BC-HIS (Board Certified

Hearing Instrument Specialist).

HIDs evaluate our hearing for the purpose of *detecting* a hearing loss and for recommending a hearing device. Among other tasks, they counsel the patient, take ear impressions, fit, set, and tune instruments. If state regulations provide for it, HIDs may also run their own business. Although many practice in retail stores, there are those who work in other areas of the hearing aid industry, such as manufacturing and sales.

It is important to know how we can verify a hearing professional's state licensure status. State health departments often maintain current licensing and certification information, which can be accessible online. Certification boards also have listings of those certified by them. Even if we do not check with official sources, we can find out a lot on our own. When going to a store, we can check if practice licenses are prominently displayed in the consultation area. We can inquire whether the vendor is an audiologist, a certified dispenser, or another clinician. We can ask if the practitioner is board certified and how long he or she has worked in the hearing device fitting and programming business. It is also important for us to evaluate whether the statements the practitioner makes regarding our hearing loss coincide with what the doctor told us. In the end, a simple conversation often tells a lot.

Determining the specialist that serves us best depends on the types of services that our hearing loss demands. In any event, we need someone with lots of practical dispensing knowledge. Two of the vendors I met along my journey had recently transitioned from manufacturing into the instrument-sales arena. They both taught me the importance of actual field experience. Matching the client with a compatible device is literally an art. It is a "fusion talent" that melds elements of science and people skills. Ultimately, the customer and the practitioner must be able to work together. If we do not like our specialist, if we feel that we are not well served, or if the personalities simply clash, the outlook for a productive outcome is grim. Overall, people cooperate poorly with professionals to whom they do not relate. When my doctor mentioned the word "compatible," I had no idea how important this would eventually be.

Federal Agencies

The Federal Trade Commission (FTC) is involved with the hearing aid world. It monitors vendor/dispenser *business practices*. It deals with issues, such as warranty and refund policy problems. It checks on activities aimed at customer deception, mostly through misleading advertising, hyped sales pitches, and inaccurate information on hearing loss or instrument performance. The FTC investigates claims of these types and can take action against the company in question.

The Food and Drug Administration (FDA) enforces regulations that target *hearing device manufacture and sale*. Hearing aids are regulated medical devices. FDA regulations specify that hearing aid practitioners must obtain a written release statement from the customer that is signed by a licensed physician. Such a certificate is to prove that the patient's hearing loss has been medically evaluated and that the patient is cleared for purchasing a hearing aid. The medical release statement cannot be older than six months.

Vendors must inform people who are found to have a hearing loss that they have to be checked out by a physician. Clients older than eighteen years of age have the right to refuse a medical evaluation and may sign a waiver to that effect. Vendors are warned, however, to advise the patient of the possible health consequences for signing such a document and to avoid encouraging people from waiving the medical check requirement. Although these regulations are meant to protect the patient, they can be difficult to enforce. Unaware of their rights, many patients shop for and obtain hearing aids without ever having seen a physician. Ethical practitioners do not let that happen. By avoiding the doctor, the question of why a person might have hearing or ear problems will not be answered, which can be dangerous for the client and bring about liability issues for the business.

This is all valuable information to keep in mind, no matter where or how we intend to buy our hearing aids.

CHAPTER 33
Buying a Hearing Aid:
Balancing Trust and Caution

Hearing aid stores are alien terrain for most of us. Overwhelmed by unfamiliar technology and tech-talk, our decisions may be based solely on the information and recommendations made by the practitioner. Certainly, hearing instrument vendors are professional people who do their best to accommodate our needs and help us to the best of their ability. Yet it is to the customer's advantage to be aware of some red flags that might pop up during the fitting and buying processes.

Not asking for a medical release statement prior to a hearing aid sale is a red flag. The same holds true for not being told about the need for a medical evaluation when a hearing loss is verified by the vendor. For reasons already amply discussed, medical checks are for the patient's protection.

Hearing aids are dispensed on a trial basis. Clients should ask about trial periods and the need for further instrument tweaking if the vendor is not forthcoming with that information. Trial periods are at least thirty days. During that time, the specialist should provide any fit or setting adjustments free of charge.

Because there are many different options on the market, qualifying for only one specific instrument is a red flag. Other choices should at least be discussed. We might wonder why the recommended device is the most appropriate one or even the only one for us. This is also a good time to discuss prices. The hearing aid that brings the most generous manufacturer incentive for the store is not necessarily the one that we can afford or that serves our needs best.

Sales pressure is yet another red flag. Are we given time to think,

261

or are we slammed through the steps? We should not buy in haste or sign documents then and there. Even during sales events, we should be able to review paperwork details in peace. It is important for us to understand the terms and conditions of the purchase agreement, warranties, and post-sale service. We must also be clear on trial periods, down-payment requirements, and possible refund policies. Whether "oral agreements" are binding is a matter for lawyers to debate but *we must get everything in writing.*

Playing Our Part - To a Point

Although the hearing aid expert is important to a successful outcome, patients also have a part in the fitting and programming processes; our input and cooperation are not only welcome but necessary. As audiologist Denise had already advised me, clinicians are guided by the tracings of our audiograms, but fitting, setting, and tuning a hearing aid is an interactive process. "How does it feel?" and "How does it sound?" are important questions that we must answer as clearly and precisely as possible. Also, patience is a virtue. Every tweak comes with an adjustment period to allow the brain to get used to the new hearing. Ideally, best results are obtained over time.

However, it is equally important to recognize when we are not moving in the right direction, no matter how many times we have returned for adjustments. Shortly after meeting with Denise, I had an experience where the settings on my mini BTE became more distorted with every visit. I never got a coherent explanation why real-ear measures were not done the way they had been explained to me in my Hearing Aid 101 class. I liked the instrument. I loved the remote control. The store was close to my house, which alleviated travel frustration, but it did not work out for me.

The time comes when we must step back and look at the overall picture. Is the recommended instrument appropriate for our hearing loss? Is the specialist's field experience sufficient for our needs? A very sophisticated and expensive digital instrument can perform dismally due to improper fitting and programming techniques. At some point, before the trial period is over, it is wise to switch clinics and seek another opinion.

Expectation Management and Careful Shopping

Of course, as hearing-aid users we want superior hearing from miracle technology in an invisible device at an attractive price. Camouflage is the key word. Downsizing hearing aids and making them more cosmetically pleasing have greatly increased their acceptability. Many reluctant customers are now willing to give better hearing a try. That is wonderful, but it is still important to manage our expectations.

It is easy to become fixated on the size of the device. In reality, the latest miniature models may not be able to accommodate the amount and type of correction that we need. Also, the smaller the instrument is, the more fragile it is, and the harder it is to manipulate. Clients with reduced finger dexterity, who have a hard time handling tiny devices and even tinier batteries, might do better with a larger hearing aid that is physically manageable and a bit more durable. Breaks and repairs are costly.

Comfort counts, too. An instrument might be "invisible," but it is of little use if it is uncomfortable to wear. Clients tend to relegate their hearing gadget to the sock drawer because they can't tolerate it—it itches, dislocates itself constantly, or feels like a thumb in the ear.

Denise had already cautioned me to read all contracts, sales agreements, and warranties. Yet vendors may also encourage customers to buy *hearing aid insurance*. Although it is important to protect one's investment, it pays to read the specifics of such policies. Different grades of coverage are offered, in plans that range from basic to premium. To avoid surprises, it is necessary for us to understand what types of extras the insurance will cover that the manufacturer warranty and store contract exclude. Usually, mishaps like snapped

RIC wires or injury resulting from crashes to the floor or the dog chomping on the device do not fit the definition of "normal wear and tear." Will the insurance pay? The terms related to "damage repair" must be clarified. How is "accidental damage" defined? Other common concerns are loss, theft, routine maintenance checks, and cleanings. It is important to be clear on when the insurance will pick up the tab. In the end, it is left for patients to review and compare the details and to decide whether insurance is worth the money. In a support meeting, a gentleman mentioned that a rider added to his home insurance policy provides comprehensive coverage for his hearing aids.

Hearing Aid Price

Although hearing instruments can have loads of features, we owe it to ourselves to inquire about all the extras with the hearing device expert. Do we really need the latest in sophistication? Some of the new, highly advanced digital hearing aids can set us back a few thousand dollars *per ear*. No wonder that the often hefty prices are cited as major obstacles to buying hearing aids. For many, cost is a huge issue. So far, we do not get financial help from most average insurance plans or from Medicare.

We are often told that hearing aid prices are bundled. This means that they do not only include the cost of the device but also all of the other services that come with the sale: hearing test, setting and tuning of the hearing aid during the trial period, maybe extra follow-up checks/adjustments and batteries as well as Aural Rehabilitation. But do we get all of these services? This is where patients and practitioners can have disagreements.

Aural rehabilitation is a comprehensive care approach that helps the hearing-challenged get the most benefit from hearing aids, assistive devices, and implants. The plan includes education about people's degree and type of hearing loss, treatment choices, advantages and limits of different hearing instruments together with communication and coping skills. The general idea is to help people adjust to their new realities through education and support. As hearing loss is a family affair, family members are also encouraged to attend aural rehabilitation sessions so that they too can learn about the diverse challenges of hearing loss and understand how important their support is.

One way to get a feel for the retail price of a certain device is to comparison shop. I was interested in a particular brand RIC digital hearing aid. I checked price listings online and called a couple of clinics at random for price quotes, which gave me an idea what the charge might be. The first available appointment was at a nearby hearing store. I was astonished when the vendor ended up asking for $800 more than the average quote. The price was scribbled on a blank piece of paper—nothing official. Obviously, my trust level hit rock bottom. The practitioner used my year-old audiogram that had been done at my last doctor visit. My hearing was never retested, as promised, and no extra services were offered to warrant such a price discrepancy. Had I not checked ahead of time, I might have paid the amount, not knowing any better. In general, I don't mind paying a bit extra for exceptional competence and attention, but at that price I expect miracles and a glass of Champagne with every visit.

That said, the high prices of digital hearing aids have led to alternatives to conventional stores and online hearing aid shopping has exploded. So, what about the need for hearing tests and medical referrals? What happens if the device needs fixing or adjusting? Does the online vendor have a local representative? Do State consumer rights still apply? These are all good questions, many without clear answers. Meanwhile, as do-it-yourself audiology seems to be taking off, I still need all the "live" professional help I can get.

Special! Special! Open House

Special One Time Offer!!!	**HURRY!**
TROUBLE UNDERSTANDING	**Hearing**
IN BACKGROUND NOISE???	**Aid**
Now Hear Every Word!	**Sale**
Free Hearing Test	**50%**
First 20 Customers	**OFF!**

Such hearing aid ads get me all conflicted. On one hand, hearing practitioners tell me to understand that hearing aids are not magic, not a fix, and that my hearing will never be the same. On the other hand, industry and store advertising almost makes me feel as if their merchandise will show me the way to hearing bliss. It might be a bit sobering, but it is important to keep both feet on the ground and not forget that *hearing loss is big business*. Ads are made to sound enticing because their goal is to get us hooked. In the hearing aid world, they are mostly used to publicize open-house promotional sales. The rather fetching message infused into most advertising is that we can get a lot of sound quality at rock-bottom prices.

However, do read the fine print. Ads often include information on the degree of hearing loss that the on-sale ware accommodates. Is that even within your range? Also, what is being sold? New and improved technology or is this a chance to sell off products that have not proven to be market successes or that are no longer considered top of the line. Is the sale device better than what you have? There is nothing wrong with hearing aid "specials." They do bring the opportunity for better hearing within reach of those who otherwise cannot afford it. However, clients will spend a still appreciable chunk of cash while their options are limited to the discounted devices that might not meet their needs.

Experienced hearing loss customers will know how to balance frugality with optimum hearing help. Sales can offer attractive deals to those who understand the hearing aid features that are helpful for their type of hearing loss and who want to upgrade their instrument or change to a different model.

Promotional ads often inform us that "manufacturer-trained specialists" will be on hand. Usually, they are involved with demonstrations and with answering questions. If they get busy testing and fitting patients, we might inquire if they are authorized to practice in our state and check on credentials.

For people who suspect or know that they have a hearing deficit but have never been checked out by a medical specialist, a sales event is not the ideal introduction to the realities of hearing loss and hearing aids. It is too easy to make plenty of misguided and uninformed decisions. Should a decline be detected during the free hearing check, the temptation is great to act on the spot and to *waive* the requirement for a formal medical evaluation in order to take advantage of the limited-time prices.

Medically cleared, first-time buyers also must be cautious. The purchase of a hearing aid is confusing even under the most relaxed of circumstances. Most novices are not yet savvy enough to make wise decisions. Charmed by the bargain, they too fail to clarify how much technology they actually need and to check on the features of competing devices. They pass on getting a second opinion regarding instrument choices and neglect to compare prices, study the paperwork, and check on the fine print.

For those who worry about having missed a chance at big savings, there will be another special in the not-so-distant future. Meanwhile, the waiting period might be used wisely to learn about the details of one's hearing loss and for collecting information on hearing aid technologies, styles, and manufacturers. Before long, the next opportunity for hearing aid bargains is upon us, and we are again in luck. Hear ye, hear ye! Open house.

PART FIVE
ASSISTIVE LISTENING; ASL;
SPEECH READING

Chapter 34
Assistive Listening Devices (ALDs)
and Applications

Assistive Listening Devices (ALDs)

Assistive listening devices help boost hearing ability, mostly through amplification. As those with hearing loss know, louder is not necessarily better, and cranking the volume up too high on an ALD, or on any device, can lead to further hearing damage. It is always best to check with the hearing specialist on additional or alternative technology that might help in different situations, such as watching TV, listening to music or participating in conversations at home or at work. In the world of ALDs, the choices are many and varied and some options can be a bit pricey.

One of most popular and useful ALD is the amplified telephone, one of the first purchases for many people with hearing loss. "Captioned" phones that display the transcribed version of a conversation on screens have pretty much replaced the paper print-outs, commonly known as TTY. The latest is the videophone for direct interaction between people using sign language or for conversations (via a relay sign language interpreter) between a hearing and a deaf or hard-of-hearing caller.

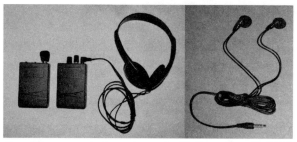

Ear phones or ear buds can be used with the pocket-sized FM Assistive Listening Device shown on the left. *photos: R.Hammond*

An ALD that probably has saved many a family dinner is a battery-operated, electronically improved, personal FM microphone/amplifier unit. About as large as a pack of cigarettes, it fits into a shirt breast pocket. It can be handheld or placed on a desk during meetings in the not-so-large office or on the table for small family dinners. It works well for one-on-one conversations. It connects to headphones and earbuds, and also plugs into other sound sources like the TV. This type of ALD is still an affordable, first-step solution for people who do not want to invest in hearing aids but who like to stay in touch with their families and friends. My mother-in-law loved hers and always took it along when she went to play Bridge with the "girls." For a hard-of-hearing relative or friend, it might make a great holiday gift. The thought of being included in the conversation could easily generate more enthusiasm than yet more bathrobes or indoor grills. Of course, it all depends on the person. The device is visible and therefore may be unacceptable to those who are fixated on hiding or denying their hearing loss.

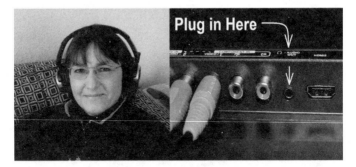

Author watches TV using noise-cancelling headphones plugged into the TV set. Audio connection detail is on the right. *photo: R.Hammond*

When I am by myself, I love to watch television or DVDs while wearing noise-cancelling headphones. They plug into the audio system and with the TV on "mute," I can listen at a volume that is comfortable.

Without background noise, the whole experience becomes more enjoyable and far less tiring.

Another gadget that I like quite a bit is my infrared (IR) TV listening device. Popular and affordable, these are sold in many different designs. People with hearing loss tend to crank up the TV volume to the point where it is intolerable to those around them. The whole neighborhood always knew which program my dad was watching—by himself as the rest of us fled.

The IR transmitter/battery-charger unit plugs into the TV. I wear a small black box, which houses the receiver/amplifier, on a neck string. Earphones or earbuds connect to this device. I adjust the volume manually. Mostly, though, I have the option of "balancing" the sound for each ear. What fascinates me is that I can put the TV and the surround-sound on mute and still listen to a program. Only I hear anything. My husband can sit in the same room and work without being bothered.

Because IR signals bounce around the room, the sound is still audible, even though I turn my back to the television while I clean or attend to my e-mail. Unlike FM systems, IR devices are only good for "line of sight" situations. The signal is interrupted by obstacles such as walls or people standing between the transmitter and the receiver. Now I can honestly inform those who step between me and my IR unit that they are truly not made of air.

For overall "louder" hearing, *very basic sound amplifiers* are sold in every electronics store as well as online. These are essentially battery-operated, no-frills, portable or in-the-ear microphones with manual volume controls. They are inexpensive, but the sound is not refined, and background noise is not attenuated.

Mostly available online or through catalogs, the upgraded, electronically more sophisticated versions of these basic devices are often called *PSAPs*, or Personal Sound Amplification Products. In ads they are also referred to as "assistive listening devices," or as "reading glasses for the ear." They might look like a Bluetooth ear piece or a behind-the-ear or in-the-ear hearing aid, which tends to confuse the consumer. These are *not* hearing aids or FDA-approved and regulated medical devices. They cannot be programmed to fit a person's specific hearing loss, and are not meant to treat hearing loss. However, depending on the product, the various sound manipulating capabilities of more upgraded versions are said to offer some help, especially to those who cannot afford regular hearing aids.

Assistive Listening Applications and Features

Nowadays, special "apps" can give smartphones frequency-tuned assistive listening capabilities. The app allows the user to adjust frequencies for clearer hearing. Want more bass, more treble? One sets it all oneself.

Although hearing aids are technically not included among ALDs, they too can benefit from a variety of assistive applications or features that further expand their usefulness for improved hearing. As we have seen, select hearing aid models can be fitted with a direct audio input (DAI) for sound access from a variety of sources. Hearing aid *Bluetooth* compatibility is a sought-after application for cell phone use, and wireless hearing aid features—especially for the purpose of "streaming"—have almost become required fare. Although they may add to the price, people who shop for hearing aids do well to inquire about the extra assistive options that different devices offer. This all shows that hearing technology offers many welcome yet complex choices. Becoming somewhat of a techie is almost inevitable.

Telecoils, together with hearing/induction loops, make up assistive listening systems that help people with hearing loss hear more clearly—especially in background noise. To be effective, the telecoil needs the loop and vice-versa. One without the other is worthless.

In general, telecoils are wireless antennas that are manufacturer-installed in hearing instruments roomy enough to accommodate them. The coil uses magnetic energy fields generated by an electrical-wire loop to bring crisper sound to hearing-assisted people. It pays to get informed on this technology as we endeavor to put loops throughout the United States.

Telecoils or T-coils

These *assistive listening features* are known by many different names—telecoil, T-coil, telephone coil, T-switch, audio coil or induction coil. The most popular and easy terms to remember are T-coil or telecoil, and they will be used throughout this text.

People with analog hearing technology already know about this feature. It was originally designed to improve telephone use for those with hearing aids. The person heard more clearly, and feedback squeals that made conversations just about impossible in the early days were much improved.

I found out quite by chance about this understated gadget called a telecoil. The topic never came up—not even during my hearing-aid training class. Like me, many hearing device clients also do not know about it. Although manufacturer-installed in many hearing aids, vendors often do not talk about it. As customers, however, we deserve to be informed.

At the start of my first support group meeting, the facilitator asked if we had switched our hearing aids into "T-coil mode." I wondered what that meant. I had never heard the expression. As the meeting progressed, I could not hear much. The fact that the speaker spoke into a microphone did not seem to help. The sound volume was too low in the room. Why didn't anyone speak up to say that the loudspeaker system did not work? Luckily, a lady sat up front with a funny little typing machine, not unlike those that are used in courts of law for taking down depositions. She transcribed every word that was said in the room onto a big screen. At least I could read and follow what went on in the meeting. I found out later on that the lady, who for two hours straight "heard" for all of us, was from the CART service—this stands for "Communication Access Real time Translation." CART is an *assistive service* that makes our meetings accessible to people with different degrees of hearing loss and to those who do not have telecoils.

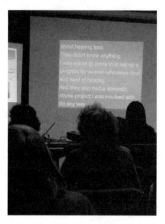

CART (Communication Access Real time - Translation) helps those who might not hear well in meetings follow the discussion word for word on the screen.
photo: R.Hammond

At the end of the session I inquired why the loudspeaker system did not work. I was told that the room was "looped." The microphones were *not* connected to a PA system but to a looping set-up. Most people at the meeting listened via telecoil, a device that makes hearing clearer and less stressful.

I wondered if my device was T-coil-enabled. No, it was not. There was no activator switch on the back of the instrument. Besides, the vented CIC was too small for housing a coil. Although they are miniaturized and refined like everything else that fits into hearing aids, telecoils still take up space in the device's shell. People who are interested in the technology must ask the vendor which hearing aids already include manufacturer-installed T-coils and then have them *activated*. That way, they can be switched on by the customers whenever they are in a "looped environment" for clearer hearing and understanding of speech.

I was a bit upset that I had not been told about the existence and advantages of such a feature. I might have chosen a different instrument style, had I only known. In addition to their not being told about telecoils, not being instructed in their proper use becomes swiftly another sore point with clients. In order to extract the best performance from the device, every T-coil must come with a training session, so that the patient understands how to use it, when and where to use it, how to switch it on, and what it can and cannot deliver.

It must also be stressed, however, that many hearing professionals believe that a T-coil should be standard equipment for those hearing aids capable of accommodating one. They also feel that a telecoil option should at least be discussed with everybody seeking hearing assistance. Many of us certainly second that opinion.

Although I do have a T-coil now, at the time I was deprived of the sound advantages that the gadget could provide. Luckily, my husband found a telecoil-equipped *portable* instrument at a specialized sound store. It has a manual volume control wheel, and it plugs into a standard set of headphones or earbuds. In microphone (M) mode, it catches sound from a loudspeaker system; in telecoil (T) mode, it taps into hearing loops. By switching the appliance to (T) mode, listening to speakers became indeed a lot less strenuous. Even though the signal was not adjusted for my hearing loss, the difference in clarity was still huge. The focus was on the voice, while background clatter was eliminated. Telecoils are not only an economical addition to boost sound quality for hearing-assisted users, they also work quite well to decrease the "listening effort" that can be so tiring and wearing on those with hearing loss.

WHAT DID YOU SAY?

Cellphone Compatibility

When buying a cellphone, it is important to check on its *hearing aid compatible* (HAC) features and sound quality at the time of purchase. As cellphone-generated radio frequency (RF) emissions can cause interference with hearing aids, the phones are given a microphone/telecoil (M/T) rating to guide the buyer. This rating assesses the potential for interference when the hearing aid is in "microphone" (M) or "telecoil" (T) mode. The lowest compatibility rating is M1/T1, while the best rating is M4/T4. The higher the rating the better the cellphone will perform whether the hearing aid is in microphone (M) or telecoil (T) mode. Clearer sound and conversations are the rewards of such favorable ratings.

Are T-coils New Technology? How Do They Work?

Even though the telecoil has been thrust into the twenty-first century, it actually has been around since the 1940s. At that time, its major job was to allow people with analog hearing aids have clearer telephone conversations, hence the name "tele-coil." In those days, phone sound was not particularly clear or loud. Also, background noise and static crackling made for poor reception under the best of circumstances. People with hearing loss had to turn their devices up, which of course resulted in bone-piercing feedback squeaks. The advent of the T-coil marked a massive communication improvement for hearing aid users. Today, it still serves its original purpose, but its role has been vastly expanded.

A telecoil is made of a very thin copper wire that coils tightly around a tiny piece of metal. The principle by which it works has its roots in the laws of physics that deal with electromagnetic fields (EMFs). The interaction of these two forms of energy—electricity and magnetism—was described ever so eloquently back in the late 1800s by Scottish mathematician and physicist James C. Maxwell. In order to apply the EMF concept to benefit people with hearing aids, somebody was really thinking outside of the box.

In short, whenever electricity flows through a wire, it generates an accompanying magnetic field that surrounds the electrical wire like an invisible expanded energy sleeve. The hearing aid T-coil dips into that magnetic field. The magnetic energy "induces" an electrical current in the coil (induction coil). This current passes through the hearing aid and on to the receiver, where it is reconverted into audible sound. The trick is that the T-coil does not respond to sound waves. Instead, it feeds on magnetic energy. The end result is that one *hears and understands speech much more clearly, especially in background noise.*

When the hearing aid is switched to T-mode, the aid's microphone is automatically turned off, which eliminates surrounding din that the microphone would otherwise pick up. However, some hearing instruments offer an M/T switch. In this mode *both* the telecoil and the hearing aid microphone are engaged. In certain situations, one might not want to be totally disconnected from the ambient noises.

T-coils Are Amazing But Not Perfect

Although telecoils have gotten a technology make-over, they are not perfect. As a hard-of-hearing person, I have stricken the word "perfect" from my vocabulary. It has been replaced by "as good as it gets."

I found out quickly that the telecoil reception is often positional, or directional. I may have to move the portable unit around a bit or tilt my head—now that I have a T-coil in my hearing aid—until I capture the cleanest, strongest signal. Telephone users know that slight rotations of the receiver may be necessary in order to get the best telecoil reception. Poorly designed hearing loops can create "dead" zones where the T-coil does not receive a signal. In that case, one has to change seats until one   reconnects with a "live" zone.

The direction of the electrical flow determines the orientation of the magnetic field. This is why the telecoil's *configuration or orientation* in the hearing aid is important. It must be in optimum "tapping" position. If we use the T-coil mostly for telephone work, it is best oriented horizontally. If we use it in looped environments, such as our meeting room, a vertical orientation is preferred. Maybe omni-directional coils will be able to alleviate such position issues in the future.

When in use, T-coils can pick up interference from other surrounding energy sources. Getting too close to computer monitors, TVs, mechanical equipment rooms or fluorescent lights, to only name a few, may result in an annoying hum or buzz. Moving away from the source can be helpful.

Moving On Up

Clearly, the telecoil has undergone some hefty makeovers in its existence. From being a simple passive coil that could not do much on its own, the device can now be programmed by the audiologist. Experts recommend, however, that T-coil settings, just as hearing aid settings, be verified with real-ear measurements.

Older coils were physically more robust than those that have to fit into ever-smaller instruments. Shrinking size means that the signal weakens also. In order to overcome that obstacle, telecoils are pre-amplified for an additional sound boost. The coil is no longer passive. It has been revamped to be quite active indeed. New and improved, the humble coil has conquered the bastion of modern-day hearing assistance: the cochlear implant, where it is standard equipment.

Induction Looping

For the T-coil to tap into a magnetic field, one must first install an electrical wire "loop" around the area that is to be made accessible. For our meetings, we have switched from a temporary loop to a permanent, professionally-installed loop.

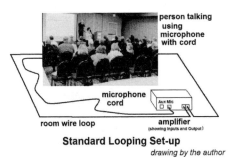

Standard Looping Set-up
drawing by the author

Hearing Loop set-up with microphone attached to cable/cord.

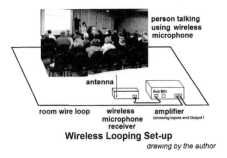

Wireless Looping Set-up
drawing by the author

Hearing Loop set-up with wireless microphone.

The basic looping system has three essential parts: a sound source—in our case, a speaker with a microphone—a special amplifier to *boost electrical current*, and an electrical wire—the loop. The wire is laid around the perimeter of the meeting room and is plugged into the amplifier. The chairs are arranged inside the area outlined by the wire. The sound source, like our microphone, connects either wirelessly to the amplifier or by means of a standard cable.

Let's say that we have a microphone with a cable attachment. The cable is plugged into the amplifier. The speaker talks into the microphone. The microphone picks up the sound energy of the voice and converts it into an electrical current. This current flows through the microphone cable to the amplifier for reinforcement. The now-

281

stronger electrical signal exits the amplifier and travels around the room, following the pre-laid wire loop. As the current flows, an accompanying magnetic field is generated around the wire. We now have created the conditions necessary for T-coil use; namely, magnetic energy. As we have already seen, the T-coil taps into the magnetic field, which *induces* an electrical current in the coil. The coil current is adjusted by the hearing aid and fed to the hearing aid's receiver, which translates the electrical signal back into audible sound. I call this awesome. The combination of induction loop and telecoil is indeed an effective assistive listening strategy for people with hearing loss.

Incidentally, the loop sound source can be anything that we want to listen to. I met a gentleman who had his den permanently looped. Now he listens through his T-coils to the TV, stereo, or computer. Wisely, he had the job professionally done. He said that he needed somebody who knew exactly what types of equipment and adapters to use and who was familiar with what plugged in to where. After all, the purpose was to hear more clearly, not to burn down the house or fry the home entertainment center.

Loop Installation

Although basic looping technology works according to the principles described earlier, it is not all that simple. Indeed, it takes savvy and specialized training to become a *certified loop installer*. For consistent signal quality, loops must conform to International Electrotechnical Commission (IEC) Standard 60118-4. They must also be integrated with other audio-visual equipment at the site, without causing interference or distortion.

When considering the installation of a hearing loop, it is important to consult with an experienced loop professional. Asking for references and certification credentials is highly recommended. After all, the success of the project depends on his/her expertise. Loop experts assess the construction features of the area to be looped. They understand client needs and budget concerns. They deal efficiently with dead zones, hums, and privacy issues due to energy spills. Most of all, they vouch for the materials that are used and stand behind their work. At the end of the job, they furnish a certificate of compliance with IEC Standards. The site www. hearingloop.org/vendors.htm displays a list of national companies involved with assistive listening loop sales and installation.

Because of the relative ease and affordability of the technology, loop systems have become quite popular for making a variety of places accessible to people with T-coil-enabled hearing devices. Overseas governments have been quick to grasp the potential public health cost savings realized through telecoils and loop systems. They determined that offering opportunities for T-coil use is a relatively inexpensive way to help people with hearing loss remain independent and socially connected. The general trend is to put the coils into public-funded hearing aids and to loop the environment. Museums, city buses, tour buses, trains, waiting rooms, information desks, bank teller and ticket windows, places of worship, and public venues are commonly looped. In London, even taxicabs are looped. In the United States, interest in the benefits of hearing loops is on a sharp rise. As people learn more, they ask—or should ask—for loop accommodation. This is after all *a matter of access*. The list of looped places is growing steadily and now includes the Chambers of the United States Supreme Court in Washington, D.C.

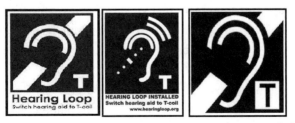

How can one tell if a place is "looped?" Watch for these signs - usually blue-and-white - marked with a prominent T. *From: LoopMinnesota, nidcd-nih-gov, napc.org*

The Neckloop

How can T-coils be used outside of a looped area? Well, we can loop ourselves by means of a "neckloop." The basic neckloop is a wire that is worn loosely around the neck. It has a tip that connects to the device to which we want to listen. Once the sound source is activated, electrical current flows through the neck wire. A magnetic field forms around the wire, into which the T-coils tap for easy listening.

Neckloops vary from the very simple to the complex. When buying such a system, it is important to get the right kind for the right purposes. The key word is "compatibility." Neckloops often specify with which types or brands of appliances a particular loop can be used. Some are meant for telephone use, while others connect to computers, MP3 players or other audio equipment. Some run on batteries and are outfitted with a volume control and even a microphone for picking up a speaker's voice—a miniature version of our meeting room set-up. This works well for one-on-one conversations or for meetings in smaller offices.

A neckloop is not just a simple piece of wire anymore. Due to the multitude of designs and configurations, it is important for us to consult the communication specialist to get an appropriate loop for our needs.

Getting Help With ALDs

When purchasing ALDs, it is best to consult a specialist who can set us up with equipment that we need, that works with what we already have, and that will truly help us. Another advantage to getting help is that we learn how to use the devices correctly. Suddenly, a plug is not a plug anymore.

When doing our own research, paging through catalogs or surfing online, we must read *all* of the product information. Some of the listed items might look wonderful, but they can be used only with specific instruments or brands. If there are specialized communication stores or distributors in our area, it pays to stop in for a consult and demonstration with an expert. Maybe what we think that we need is not the best choice. There could be a more practical or a cheaper way. Personally, I like to see and feel what I buy. I want to know what the device looks like, sounds like, feels like, and how much it weighs. I want to know if I need an engineering degree in order to operate it. I want to know where the adjustment knobs are and how easy they are to reach and handle. I want to check if changing the batteries will become a family effort.

Chapter 35
American Sign Language (ASL) and Speech Reading

American Sign Language

Throughout time, hand signs were used as a way of communicating when silence was of the essence. In religious orders where talking was not allowed, hand signals commonly relayed information or allowed for "chatting" on the sly. On military missions non-verbal sign communication is used to keep one's position and presence from being revealed.

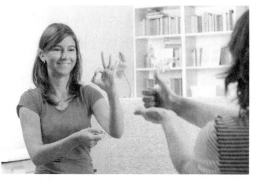

"Signing" is the language of deaf and/or severely hearing-challenged people.
photo: (c) Amaviael www.fotosearch.com

"Signing" is the language of hearing-challenged people for whom hearing assistance is of little or no help and who often refer to themselves as "deaf." It is also the primary language of people who are born deaf. Across the world, signing differs from country to country. By choosing the most relevant and easily understood signs from various sign languages, an international signing system has been established. International Sign (IS) facilitates deaf communication worldwide. It is mostly used for conferences, athletic events, or fairs that people from different nations attend. In the United States, we use American Sign Language (ASL). Communication between hearing people and those who sign is facilitated by ASL interpreters. Interpreters often specialize in different areas, such as legal, business, education, or medical signing.

In many states students can fulfill their second language requirement with sign language. Learning ASL, however, is a very dynamic process. There is a lot more to it than just signing. Lip motions allow for speech-reading, while facial expressions and body language combine with the hand signs. Together, they convey the feeling and context that a verbal speaker projects through voice manipulations, such as variations in loudness, pitch, and tone. What is true for spoken languages is also true for ASL. The earlier one starts signing, the better it is, and perfection comes to those who persevere. Ongoing practice with a fluent signer is a must if one wants to keep the skill alive.

ASL courses are taught across the country. Local school districts usually offer a variety of venues and times from which to choose. My classes were heavily attended by hearing people who wanted to communicate with deaf relatives or friends. Many were grandparents in search of ways to connect with a deaf grandchild. As I set out to study ASL, I found that this is a complicated language to learn. Grammar is signed. The sentence structure is different from spoken English. Limited finger dexterity and vision issues can become problems for "mature" students. I had a hard time separating the actual signs from finger-spelling that is used for names or words that do not have a sign. Reading the alphabet in mirror image at mach speed also had its challenges. I acquired a great respect for proficient signers.

In general, those who have lost their acoustic hearing over time—or suddenly, like me—do not sign. Hard-of-hearing (HOH) people tend to resist ASL until assistive hearing technology is no longer an option. Many, if not most of my HOH friends, however, know at least some basic signs. Yet to follow or carry on conversations, a person must be quite fluent in ASL or the help of interpreters is needed. Although it is hard to achieve perfection, as hard-of-hearing people we should be energized by the thought that every sign that we learn works to our advantage as we journey through the world of hearing loss.

Speech Reading

Speech reading is often referred to as "lip-reading." It is a technique for recognizing sounds or words by the movements of the tongue and by the shape of the speaker's lips. Speech reading is a skill that takes years to learn and to perfect, up to a point. Yet we all do a bit of this, especially under challenging communication circumstances such as noisy environments. We observe people's mouths trying to confirm that what we hear is accurate. For hearing-challenged people, speech reading is an essential tool for following a conversation, particularly if it is used in combination with other cues such as facial expressions and body language. Yet only about 30 to 40 percent of English language sounds are visible and their correct identification is further complicated because many have identical mouth positions. Is it bet or pet?

In view of these difficulties, we should not expect those with hearing loss to read every word right from our lips. Speech reading works best for one-on-one conversations in quiet, well-lit settings where the speaker and the "reader" have each other's attention and face one another. Even the most skilled speech readers cannot determine what was said if people keep turning their heads, laugh while they talk, or talk with food in their mouths. Mustaches and beards that hide lip features also hinder speech reading.

Communicating with Hard-of-Hearing People

When communicating with hard-of-hearing or deaf people, it is important

- to get the person's attention first
- to face the conversation partner
- to speak calmly and distinctly at a voice level that is comfortable for the hard-of-hearing person
- to avoid interrupting conversations
- to avoid speaking through barriers, such as doors or walls
- to remember that once hard-of-hearing or deaf people are not in the speaker's direct line of sight, they are also out of "earshot," no matter how physically close they may be.

PART SIX
SURGICAL IMPLANTS

Chapter 36
Hearing Device Implants

Once considered a rarity, ultra-high-tech implantable systems are now produced by a variety of manufacturers. Every company has a different, patented approach for helping people with types and degrees of hearing loss that were once considered untreatable. Although such devices do not fix hearing loss, they offer the patient a chance for boosted hearing, better understanding of speech, and improved sound perception.

Before any implantation can be considered, the patient will be screened by a team of experts, which includes ear surgeons, audiologists, nurses, and anesthesiologists. They review the results of ear exams, scans, and hearing tests. They evaluate the patient's health and hearing histories and perform the necessary pre-surgical medical assessments. They interview the patient and explain the details of the procedure, anesthesia, surgical risks, possible complications, and post-surgery care. They also address the truths and myths surrounding the implant and answer any questions. Financial details are evaluated by insurance specialists.

As this can be a bit overwhelming, it is advisable to bring a friend or family member to the appointments to help the patient formulate questions, lend support, and collect information. Ultimately, the implant experts decide if the preset criteria have been met. If so, the surgery will be eventually performed at an implant-accredited surgical center.

I do not qualify for any of these devices and do not endorse one instrument or manufacturer over another. However, I believe that all people with hearing loss should have at least some knowledge of how implants are meant to work. Although technology changes and improves at lightning speed, I endeavor to describe the basics of those implants that are currently on the market.

Chapter 37
Middle Ear Implants (MEIs)

Middle ear implants are meant to assist people with sensorineural hearing loss who have not been helped by conventional hearing aids or who cannot tolerate them. The advantage is that middle ear implants leave the ear canal totally open. No more itching. No more tubes and anchor buds. No more feedback. No more occlusion. Candidates are evaluated by an implant team to assure that they meet the criteria for the procedure and for best hearing results.

Manufacturers have their own electronic recipes and trademark designs for making these instruments most efficient. The main issue is to reinforce the mechanical signal that is transferred to the cochlea by increasing ossicle vibration directly. Vibrations can be enhanced or slowed according to the patient's hearing requirements. A crucial feature of the surgical procedure is the installation of electronic parts onto the ossicle chain of the middle ear. Currently, there are two MEI editions available in the United States: a semi-implant and a full implant.

The *semi-implanted* device has both internal and external parts. A battery-operated and microphone-equipped sound processor is worn unobtrusively in back of the ear. It connects magnetically and wirelessly through the skin to the two-component implanted portion of the system. The processor's microphone picks up outside sounds and changes them into electrical signals, which are transmitted through the skin to the receiver of the implanted prosthesis. From the receiver, the signals travel to the ossicle-mounted transducer, which converts electricity back into vibrations that stimulate the ossicle chain. Ultimately, the stapes transmits the vibrations to the inner ear.

The cochlear hair cells change the vibrations to electrical impulses that travel to the brain via the cochlear nerve. After the surgical wound has healed, the patient is fitted with the external processor that is programmed by the audiologist according to the patient's hearing needs.

The *fully implanted* device is three-component system. There are no external parts; even the battery is implanted. The implant does not have a microphone. Instead, the ear itself is its own natural microphone. In order to capture the sound in the most efficient way, the outer ear, ear canal, and eardrum must be in good condition. Normal function of the eustachian tube is also required.

Natural sound vibrations from the eardrum and ossicles are picked up by an internal sensor, which converts the mechanical vibration energy into an electrical current. The current then passes through a sound processor, where it is amplified and adjusted according the patient's hearing needs. From the processor, the tuned electrical signal moves on to a driver which changes it back into vibrations that vibrate the stapes. The stapes transmits the vibrations to the cochlea of the inner ear. The user can turn the device on and off or adjust the volume by means of a remote control device.

Depending on usage, the implanted battery can last for years. A light indicates when the battery is running low. Battery replacement is done under sedation and local anesthesia during a short surgical procedure.

Chapter 38
Cochlear Implants and
Auditory Brainstem Implants (ABI)

Cochlear Implant (CI)

Just as hearing aids have undergone considerable technological makeovers, so have cochlear implants. For centuries, researchers have been fascinated by using electrical stimulation of the ear to produce hearing. Around 1790, Italian physicist Count Alessandro Volta, who pioneered work on what we know now as a "battery," is said to have been the first person to place metal rods into his ears and to connect them to an electrical circuit. He reported getting a loud boom in his head, followed by a crackling, bubbling sound, as if some thick soup were boiling. It was not a pleasant experience, but his idea of using electricity to facilitate hearing took hold.

Since then, a long list of scientists have studied and debated the feasibility or value of electrically stimulating the hearing nerve. The question was whether this tactic might restore sound perception to deaf and profoundly hard-of-hearing people. In the 1960s, research greatly accelerated. Building on each others' victories and defeats, strings of researchers and scientists, as well as very courageous pioneer patients, led to the development of the instrument known today as a cochlear implant (CI). In the United States, the FDA approved cochlear implants for adults in 1984 and in 1990 for children.

Filling in for Cochlear Cells

A cochlear implant (CI) acts on behalf of damaged and dead cochlear cells and electrically stimulates the hearing nerve directly. Results are best if the hearing nerve is undamaged and in good working order. A CI can benefit deaf people and those with severe to profound sensorineural hearing loss when conventional hearing aids cease to be helpful.

A CI does not "fix" a hearing loss. Once the device is turned off or disconnected, the patient is back to the starting hearing level. However, when in use, it helps recapture a sensation of sound and understanding of speech. Adjusting to the implant takes time and patience. Initially, sound might appear somewhat metallic, especially to those who remember normal acoustic hearing, but after a while, it usually takes on a more natural quality.

Before getting a CI, many patients go through the "hearing aid drill" until those devices are overtaxed and no longer help. A lady told me that one of her hearing aids actually gave her headaches, yet in spite of all of the droning amplification, she heard almost nothing. Her cochlea was essentially dead. Her other ear was also weak and failing. She got a CI and claimed that she never looked back. Compared to what she had, she felt this was heaven, even though it was not perfect. On the other hand, I also have met those who had a dickens of a time getting an acceptable result. One wonders if the problems were with the surgery, the instrument, the patient's expectations, or the programming.

The most amazing statement that I have heard from various CI users is that their tinnitus either went away or improved dramatically—this would make sense. As the brain receives input from across the whole frequency spectrum, it can ease its mad search for the missing sound signals.

The CI Candidate and the Team

As described earlier, before anyone is considered for an implant, he/she must be evaluated by the "implant team." These are specialists with expertise in the *various phases* of the cochlear implant process. They tend to work with the instruments of particular manufacturers. That way they are informed about the latest upgrades and trained in the newest techniques. They evaluate the client's physical and emotional status before surgery, perform the procedure, provide after-surgery care, tune the instrument, train the patient, and continue working with him/her for best and consistent results. There are specific criteria and qualifications that the team will consider in the selection of the candidate.

The surgical procedure is only the beginning of a long journey; most of the critical work is done afterwards. Therefore, it is important that the patient is both willing and able to cooperate with audiologists and/or speech pathologists in what will be a rather lengthy rehabilitation process to retrain the brain. The recipient must be motivated and committed to the CI journey. Support from family and friends increases the chances for the venture to be a positive one.

Getting a CI is a major decision that raises many concerns for patients and family alike. Along with their questions about the procedure, the odds for success, and healing times, patients might wonder how many implants the team has done. They might also ask what action would be taken if the FDA recalled their instrument. Although this sounds extreme, it has happened. Problems and adverse events related to CIs can be reported to the FDA MedWatch program.

When meeting with the experts, the important issue is to get satisfactory answers to all questions and worries. In this complicated process, it is easy to get confused and intimidated. Yet we often ask for more information from a prospective handyman who will work in our yard than we do of our medical care providers.

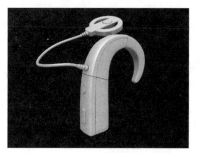

External parts of a Cochlear Implant: behind the ear processor with attached cable & antenna. Antenna connects to implanted parts via magnet.
photo: (c) dreamdesigns www.fotosearch.com

Surgery and Parts

The very delicate implant surgery is done under general anesthesia. It usually lasts about two hours, but it can be longer. Most people go home the day of surgery or the morning after, and return to work within a week. Before the implant is put into service, the surgical wound must heal, which takes four to six weeks. To increase the odds for a successful outcome, an experienced surgeon is an absolute must, as is an expert audiologist who finally sets and tunes the device. Although the systems may vary among the different manufacturers, there are commonalities, and the surgical and rehabilitation procedures are essentially the same.

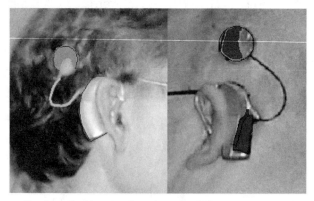

Caption: Cochlear Implants in action. *photos: R.Hammond*

A cochlear implant has both *external* and *internal* (implanted) parts. Traditionally, the *external* portion looks like a BTE hearing aid. It contains the microphone(s), sound-processing circuitry, a battery, and a T-coil. It is attached by a thin cable to a round headpiece, which is actually a transmitter antenna. A magnet embedded in the headpiece/ antenna unit connects through the skin to a magnet located on the implanted portion of the CI system.

A newer design incorporates the above-mentioned external electronics and magnets into a disc-shaped, *all-in-one* unit, which eliminates the connector cable and BTE-like piece.

The *implanted or internal* part is made of the receiver/stimulator unit and an array of ultrathin, flexible electrodes. In order to install the internal unit, the surgeon makes a cut into the skin behind the ear that will be implanted. The mastoid bone is exposed and prepared to accommodate the receiver/stimulator. The inner ear is accessed via a hole that is drilled through the mastoid bone. The electrodes are threaded into the cochlea, ever so gently. The number of electrodes varies between manufacturers. Newer devices have more than twenty. As the electrodes are assigned to different frequency ranges, the more electrodes, the better the clarity and quality of sound will be—at least in theory. Once all the parts are in position and secured, the wound is closed and allowed to heal for about four weeks.

The Long Way to the Hearing Nerve

To connect the external and implanted CI parts, either the traditional external antenna-headpiece or the all-in-one unit is positioned over the implant site, which allows the internal and external magnets to link up. Now, all parts communicate, and sound signals can travel through the skin from the external unit to the implanted electrodes. In brief, the external microphone picks up sound and converts it into electrical current. The sound processor converts the current into digital signals that it adjusts according to individual parameters programmed by the audiologist. Regardless of the external design, the adjusted signals travel through the skin to the implanted receiver. The internal receiver transfers the signals to the implanted electrodes, which relay them to the hearing nerve, which forwards them to the brain.

Activation Day and Mapping

The healing of the surgical wound takes about a month. Many patients say that this is a hard time for them. They wonder if they made the right decision or if the device will work for them after so much physical and emotional turmoil. It is certainly understandable that a person might feel both apprehensive and a bit jittery with anticipation.

Finally, the day arrives when the client sees the audiologist for the initial "hook-up" between all the parts of the CI. This is also known as "activation day," when contact between the external and implanted parts is established for the first time. It is also the first time that the patient senses sounds with the new device. There might be some scratchy noises, blips, or echoes, which are all good things, but understanding speech is still a way off. The arduous task of putting the CI online and making it fully functional has just begun.

First, the audiologist runs a series of preliminary equipment tests on the different components to make sure that all systems are in good working order. After the checks are complete, the serious job of establishing some basic settings will begin. Programming a CI is a rather lengthy process, called *mapping.* The system is like a blank canvas that has to be filled in with the parameters particular to the patient's listening needs. Setting threshold levels, comfort levels, electrical stimulation limits, and more will take a while. During the first month, several sessions are usually scheduled. The audiologist and the patient must work together as a motivated team in order to get the job done. However, mapping is never really finished; it is an ongoing process. Periodic checks and mapping adjustments are needed in order to assure the optimal performance of the CI.

Who Can Benefit from a Cochlear Implant?

Some of the adult candidates for CI implantation are patients who lost most, if not all, of their functional hearing due to severe cochlear damage. Eventually, conventional hearing aids are no longer of much help. At that point, inquiring about a CI is certainly appropriate. Both cochlear implant technology and surgical procedures have come a long way to help these people maintain quality of life by staying engaged with their families, social activities, and professional environments. The difference that a CI has made in the lives of friends who struggled for years with hearing aids and who had just about given up hope is huge.

Under FDA guidelines, babies who are born deaf or profoundly hard of hearing become CI candidates as of 12 months of age. According to statistics from the National Institute on Deafness and Other Communication Disorders (NIDCD), nine of every ten children who are born deaf in the United States are born to hearing couples. Stunned parents suddenly need a lot of unbiased information on resources that are available to help their children, as well as the family. Invariably, the cochlear implant option is seen as a way to get the children integrated into the "hearing world." Deaf parents, however, may choose to pass on the CI and to raise their child in the deaf culture.

As children are implanted, CI-hearing will become "normal hearing" to them. The expectation is that they will grow up learning to detect and identify noises and sounds, while acquiring speech capabilities that will allow them to attend mainstream schools. Although hearing parents might be eager to embrace the idea of a cochlear implant, they must remain aware of the child's ongoing severe hearing challenges. Sign language facilitates communication when the CI is off. Although it can be very helpful, the CI will not solve all communication and learning issues and a network of additional resources and support is needed for the child and the family.

As already stated, cochlear implant surgery is only the beginning of a long journey. It will take the commitment of the whole family to assist and support the child as he/she passes through testing, surgery, mapping, rehabilitation exercises, and speech therapy sessions. The family learns alongside the youngster as they explore a totally different dimension of what we know as the "sense of hearing."

Deaf people may also choose to try a CI, and many have mastered hearing and understanding speech through the implant. Yet many admit that the process is quite daunting. Being introduced rather suddenly to our world of din can be both frightening and confusing. Discovering what written and signed words might sound like has been described as challenging but exciting. Obviously, it takes therapy and plenty of patience and practice to detect, identify, and interpret the signals coming in through the CI. The challenge demands outright courage that is not to be underestimated.

***

CI Controversy in the Deaf Community

Initially, the advent of the CI stirred up great controversy and anxiety among deaf people. The fear was that the technology would become a threat to the *deaf culture,* a world that nurtured them and where they found friends and social connections when the so-called "hearing world" did not exactly embrace or help them. They also worried about becoming the targets of glossy, misleading marketing campaigns and about being pushed toward implantation. Many objected to the idea of being "fixed," while others who became intrigued by the implant option were afraid that they might be looked upon as "betraying" their own. We now know that cochlear implants are not a "cure" or a "fix" for deafness. They merely open the world of sound temporarily to the user. Once the headpiece is disconnected, so is the sound.

At the outset, however, misleading and incomplete information abounded as the CI put its mark on the hard-of-hearing world. Deaf people raised some very valid concerns regarding the procedure itself, the technology and its shortcomings, as well as the physical and emotional fallout. As more information became available and as overly optimistic statements were put through the reality checks, the deaf community worked itself through the CI issues and took the position that having or not having a CI is a matter of personal choice. While many deaf parents with deaf children decide to raise them in the deaf community the way they were brought up themselves, others may decide to give the implant a chance, especially because of potential advantages related to their children's educational opportunities.

This said, a young lady once related that education for deaf people has come a long way. Besides special schools for the deaf, there are many helpful technology resources available that did not exist just a few years back. She stated that she is quite content within the deaf community and that CI technology leaves her cold. However, she relies heavily on electronic communication devices and is very speedy at texting.

A lingering concern in the deaf community is that people who consider the option of a CI should be given relevant and complete information about the truths and the myths, the pros and the cons of implantation. They also want potential CI users to understand the facts regarding the need for special education services, sign language skills, and other support services, even in case of implantation. Yet in the end, to have or not have a CI is a decision for the individual to make.

***

Hybrid Cochlear Implant

The latest FDA-approved system is a "hybrid" implant, which combines the functions of a hearing aid with those of a cochlear implant in one device. However, the implanted portion has shorter electrodes than the conventional CI. It is meant for those who have a severe to profound hearing loss in the high frequencies but who can still hear low frequencies well enough with or without a hearing aid. The shorter electrodes do not affect the still active lower frequency

305

areas in the cochlea. If needed, the hearing aid part boosts the lower frequencies, which results in a combination of acoustic and electronic hearing.

Auditory Brainstem Implant (ABI)

What about helping those who do not qualify for cochlear implantation due to severe inner-ear abnormalities and/or hearing nerve issues? The Auditory Brainstem Implant (ABI) has been developed for this purpose. Similar in design to the cochlear implant, but different in function, the ABI also has external and implanted parts. However, the internal electrodes of this highly complex system stimulate targeted hearing areas in the *brainstem* directly—bypassing the inner ear and hearing nerve. After programming, many patients gain meaningful sound awareness, which is important for communication. Speech-reading scores often improve. Since the publication of the first edition of this book, remarkable progress in ABI technology has been made, and efforts are ongoing to further refine ABI results. As with all hearing technology, the ultimate goal is the understanding of speech and the appreciation of music.

Chapter 39
Bone-Conduction Implants

Patients with a conductive hearing loss, a mixed hearing loss or a one-sided deafness may become candidates for a bone-conduction hearing system. Although there are different designs by different manufacturers, the purpose remains the same: to bring sound vibrations to the cochlea via the skull bones. Again, specific parameters must be met in order to qualify for an implant.

Bone-anchored Hearing Aid (BAHA)

The bone-anchored hearing aid (BAHA) is a semi-implantable system that bypasses the outer and middle ear structures and relays sound vibrations directly to the cochlea. No more headbands. No more pressure and skin irritations. No more air-conduction aids that are often of little help. When compared to the head-worn instruments, the BAHA overall sound quality is said to be tremendously improved.

I have a colleague who dealt with a complicated conductive hearing loss for some time. Conventional hearing aids were better than nothing at all, but they failed to serve his needs, especially on the job. Eventually, he was evaluated for a BAHA and qualified. What a difference it made! It is wonderful to see technology work a bit of magic. Granted, his hearing is not totally perfect under every circumstance, but it is great to see him so relieved, so upbeat, and so smiley.

Screening for a BAHA

Unlike other implants, the BAHA allows for a pre-surgery trial run, which is great. If the head-worn version of the instrument improves the client's hearing, chances are that the implant will do a lot better. However, the patient must meet other qualification criteria as well. An implant team evaluates whether the applicant is indeed a good candidate for this technology. The steps of the screening process are similar to those already cited for other implants.

Audiograms and hearing and health histories are reviewed. The specialists will ask what other devices have been tried and what the client expects from the implant. Mental and physical abilities come into consideration. The patient must have enough finger dexterity to apply and remove the processor, which is both expensive and fragile. My colleague has a fine tether wire that clips to his shirt collar. Should the device come loose for whatever reason, the tether prevents it from crashing to the floor. Of course, financial details and insurance coverage realities are explored. The team educates the qualifying client on the surgical procedure and on the pros and cons of the technology. Again, the screening interview also offers the patient a perfect opportunity for questioning the specialists.

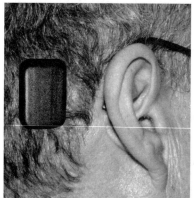

The Bone Anchored Hearing Aid (BAHA) processor sends sound vibrations to the inner ear via the skull bones. *photo: R.Hammond*

Parts and Procedure

The BAHA system has three parts: the titanium implant, the

abutment, and the sound processor. Two of these are installed during a short operation that can be done under local anesthesia. The procedure takes about an hour.

On the side of the implant, a small area of skin is shaved and prepared behind the ear. The surgeon then makes an incision, lifts a flap of skin, and exposes the mastoid bone. Then he/she drills a small hole into the bone into which the *titanium implant*—which is described as a tiny screw or stud—is secured. When put into action, the implant screw will act as the "skull bone rattler." A connector socket, called an *abutment,* is screwed into the implant stud. The abutment will protrude slightly through a slit in the skin flap that will be stitched back into place. After the healing of the surgical site is complete, the abutment is connected to the *digital sound processor.* This unit looks like a small rectangular box. It houses a battery, microphone(s), sound-processing circuitry, and an oscillator.

An updated version of this bone-anchored system is to connect the titanium implant screw to a *magnet* instead of the abutment. This implant/magnet duo is installed completely under the skin—no more protrusion. The external sound processor is also attached a magnet. Once the processor is applied to the implant site, the external and implanted parts communicate while being held magnetically in place.

Becoming One with the Bone

Healing takes two to three months. During that time, the incision heals but most importantly, bone forms around the titanium implant, which literally becomes one with the surrounding bone. This process, called *osseo-integration,* is crucial for the implant to work properly. One does not want a wobbly titanium implant. If bone integration progresses slowly, the waiting period for the processor becomes longer.

Eventually, the osseo-integration is complete. Once it is deemed acceptable by the surgeon, the patient is cleared for seeing the audiologist. Fitting and tuning of the sound processor are next.

Good Sound Vibrations

The microphone of the processor unit captures environmental sounds and changes them into electrical signals. These signals are digitized, amplified, and adjusted, according to the patient's hearing needs. They are then relayed to the processor's oscillator, which converts them into vibrations that travel—either through the abutment or the magnets—to the titanium implant. Once "rattled," the implant sets off vibrations within the skull bones that reach the cochlea of the inner ear. Here, they are translated into electrical signals that will stimulate the hearing nerve—that is the very short version. Between the capture of sound and the cochlea, a whole lot of signal refinement and translation takes place within these bone conduction instruments of the twenty-first century.

The Expanding Uses of the BAHA System

Although the bone-anchored implant was originally intended to help patients with a conductive or mixed hearing loss, its use has since been expanded. The BAHA got the nod for treating patients with a one-sided sensorineural deafness or severe to profound hearing loss, *if* the other ear tests normal or near normal. Traditionally, the "one good ear and one deaf ear" situation is vexing for the patient and presents the audiologist with a wiring or rigging challenge. When only one ear is severely affected, the patient does not hear in "stereo" anymore, which creates quite a few issues, such as difficulty understanding speech in noisy environments, equilibrium problems due to lopsided hearing, and being unable to tell the direction of sound, which as I well know is mighty annoying and even dangerous. In order to hear people who sit on their "deaf" side, clients must continuously turn the head toward the sound source.

In an attempt to provide more normalized hearing to such patients, a technique called CROS or BiCROS can be employed. Although various sources express it slightly differently, CROS stands for "contralateral routing of offside signal," which means that sound signals captured on the side of the seriously challenged or deaf ear are transferred over to the cochlea of the good ear.

For CROS, the patient has an air-conduction BTE or ITE hearing device for *each* ear. The device for the deaf side is equipped with a microphone. The device for the normal side has a receiver microphone. If the better ear has some degree of hearing loss, a hearing aid that assists the better ear while also receiving signals from the deaf side will be used. This technique is referred to as BiCROS.

On the deaf side, the microphone picks up sound and changes it into electrical signals, which are then transmitted to the normal or better hearing ear. The signal transfer between the devices can be done wirelessly, via radio signal, or by means of a physical connection, such as a wire—to which most people object. The wire may be hidden in the hair, or it can be installed onto a headband-type system, which makes for a sturdier but more visible option.

In simple terms, with a CROS or BiCROS set-up, the good ear also "hears" for the deaf ear. In a social setting it is possible to hear people who talk to us on our "bad" side. CROS/BiCROS can give the impression of more balanced hearing as the stereo sensation is restored at least to some extent. Also, many report that their sense of equilibrium is much improved.

Dealing with the CROS dilemma has become an added use for the BAHA implant. The BAHA is installed behind the impaired ear. Sound signals that are captured on the deaf side are translated into vibrations, which are relayed by bone conduction to the functioning side, where they stimulate the cochlea of the good ear. Again, the patient recovers a sensation of hearing in both ears, which helps with speech understanding and sound localization. It provides an overall feeling of normalized, stereo hearing. The BAHA provides kind of a CROS action without extra hearing instruments and other trappings.

Magnetic Bone-conduction Implant

Another bone-conduction hearing implant is a totally magnetic system—without a titanium stud. The implanted part is completely hidden under the skin. It consists of a set of two magnets that are sealed into a titanium case. The magnet plate is firmly affixed to the bone during a short surgical procedure. Once the wound has healed and inflammation has gone down, the patient can be fitted with the external sound processor, which is also equipped with a magnet. The connection between internal and external magnets keeps the processor snuggly in place. Sound vibrations adjusted for the patient's hearing are transmitted by the processor through the skin to the skull bone from where they travel to the cochlea of the inner ear.

PART SEVEN
FEELINGS and EMOTIONS, SUPPORT GROUPS and ORGANIZATIONS

Chapter 40
Feelings and Emotions

When I was first sidelined by hearing loss and tinnitus, I had no idea that a wild emotional roller coaster was awaiting me. Too much happened all at once—too much loss, too much change, and too many questions without satisfactory answers. Along with the trepidations that came with all the medical investigations, I felt buried under an avalanche of feelings, none of them good or helpful. In the end, the clinical mysteries turned out to be the more manageable part of the whole experience.

Whether it strikes suddenly or progresses stealthily and slowly, the emotional consequences of hearing loss and accompanying challenges can be overwhelming. Life is no longer the same, and lifestyle changes and adaptations are in order. Mostly, though, along with fading hearing come serious communication difficulties that tempt people to curtail their interactions with others—and that can be a set-up for social isolation, lonesomeness, and ultimately, depression.

Dealing with the consequences of my sudden losses proved to be a tall order. Even after all this time, the echoes of "that day's" events continuously remind me of the changes that forced themselves upon me, literally overnight. Gone was my effortless hearing; I now strain to listen and to understand. I squint as I try to concentrate and pay attention. I misunderstand. I do not understand. As background din drowns out voices or blends with them, it doesn't take long before I feel as if I have swirls of Bundt cake dough in my head. No matter how interesting the conversation topic is, the back-and-forth word fights of people interrupting one another and yelling in order to make a point simply wear me down. I become quiet or tune out, which is so not like me. This is when I am usually told that I am not my *"old self."*

I always loved my work and took great pride in my profession. Keeping my job became the ultimate challenge that I desperately wanted to meet. I managed to do so with difficulty for a while, but eventually my efforts ground to a halt, and I had to let go. The job was gone. Also gone was my perfect sense of balance. I now watch every step that I take. Being wobbly certainly does not pep up my self-confidence. Gone is the time when I could sit quietly and read or just enjoy a solitary moment. Tinnitus, my unrelenting ear phantom, makes sure of that.

Yes, it became easy to keep track of my losses while taking my blessings for granted. In order to heal and to find the "new me," that would have to change.

Meanwhile, I was totally overwhelmed. Even before I emerged from the fog of processing the events and from the initial medical frenzy, I realized that the road ahead was no longer straight or predictable. It abruptly wandered off into unfamiliar territory. Off-kilter with a head abuzz with tinnitus, how would I even begin to manage my new life? Would I always be this desperate and angry?

Eventually, I got this feeling of an emotional déjà vu. I remembered that way back in pharmacy college, we had studied something called the "grief cycle." Much of it could be applied to my present situation, and I actually derived quite a bit of relief from this. I was not simply a self-absorbed whiner feeling sorry for myself. On the contrary, I was slugging my way through a natural but bumpy process, side-tracked by self-doubt, fear and a generous dose of mental anguish.

The Contorted Path to Healing

In the 1960s, a Swiss doctor, Elisabeth Kübler-Ross, wrote so eloquently in her book *On Death and Dying* about the ultimate human test—death. She talks about the emotional cycles that terminally ill people pass through before they finally arrive at accepting their destiny and finding peace. The same emotional swings also apply to loss in general, whether we lose a friendship, our job, our lifestyle, our personal freedom—or our hearing.

Changes brought on by events that we see as massively negative set us up for sorrow and grief. We mourn the loss and progress through a cycle of emotions that will eventually reconcile us with the new realities and allow us to move on with our lives. Many people make the journey toward acceptance automatically and go forward, while others need professional assistance in order to overcome the obstacles that litter the way. Cycle of grief expressions, such as shock, denial, anger, depression, testing, and acceptance suddenly rang quite true with me.

Working through the issues has not been a nicely delineated process. Moving from shock to acceptance is not a neatly laid-out recipe, and it became a rough ride. I tended to bounce around a bit jostled by a whirlwind of conflicting feelings. Up and down I went. I must admit that I spent the first day after my ear event feeling numb and in a state of controlled shock. In the years that I had spent in health care, I had witnessed plenty of times when traumatic incidents struck people with disbelief so profound that it took them to the edge of emotional shut-down.

Although I was plenty distraught, I never denied the medical facts of my condition. I was in denial, however, about how my life would be affected by the limits that had been bestowed on me. I did not know what to do, and so I pretended that not that much had happened. Life goes on, right? At the cost of mental and physical exhaustion, I returned to teaching and to working at the pharmacy. I gave the impression that things were just fine. People even commented on how well I coped with the situation, which made me feel guilty. Yet I did not want to dispel the myth of my "impressive" recovery—another variation on the theme of denial. At first, I thought that keeping some normalcy in my life would be helpful. However, the notion of "normalcy" had taken on a totally new meaning.

While appearing rather serene on the outside, on the inside a massive storm was gathering strength. By and by, I became angry at fate and frustrated with myself and with the often spiritless yet hugely expensive health system that seemed to have abandoned me. I was tremendously grateful for the medical treatment that I had received, but it came up short on satisfactory answers. In order to get resolution, I needed explanations and context. My off-the-charts frustration abated somewhat when I realized that it was up to me to enlighten myself on the clinical details of my condition and on available resources.

Initial research efforts were cut short by my slow slide into a period of guilt-fueled depression. I felt guilty for being unable to cope better and faster, for wrecking everybody else's life, for not contributing financially the way I used to, especially as a stack of medical bills reminded me of my greatly reduced work schedule. I felt guilty for being so self-absorbed when my issues paled in comparison to those of so many others. I kept wondering where I had gone wrong and what I could have done differently. Instead of moving forward, such self-analysis threw me back into the past. I became an emotional wet noodle, overwhelmed by feelings of hopelessness and worthlessness.

Finding a New Reference Point

For quite a while I was stalled on the road to healing, looking back. The biggest problem was that the "old life" kept on being my reference point. Mired in the past, I threatened to become my own biggest stumbling block as I strained to move forward. No wonder that progress was slow. I forgot about an old warfare motto that advises never to surrender territory that already has been paid for in blood. The "blood" in this case was made of frustration, physical and emotional trauma, self-doubt, self-blame, and an ample amount of tears. Rather than contemplating what used to be, it was time to focus on what was to come, the new life. I had to find the "positives" and weave them into a new future. For that, however, my emotional GPS was in dire need of recalibration—the sooner, the better.

It Was Not All about Me

Meanwhile, living with me had become a challenge. One day, my husband, Ross, mentioned that, in spite of his best efforts, he really could not relate to what I was talking and obsessing about. He felt that we had to find people who could understand and relate. He said "we." That was the day that I realized that hearing loss with all of its side issues is not all about those affected, but that it is also a lot about others—family, friends, and coworkers who see them struggle, who would like to help but don't know how. I had become dismissive about all the articles sent to me that related to hearing loss, the ads clipped from magazines telling about treatments and resources. People tried to reach out, to help, and I really needed to get a grip. It was not all about me!

Ross' checking on local support groups turned out to be a major leap forward on the path to recovery. I met people who could relate. I learned a lot, as I will share a bit later, but I also received a serious compassion wake-up call and a bit of a lesson in humility, which proved to be very therapeutic.

Acceptance and Peace Within

A gradual turnaround had started earlier when our daughter found the words to frame the issue and became the voice of reason. She patiently told me that I had to quit the self-torture and become kinder and more forgiving toward myself. I hadn't special-ordered these difficulties, she reminded me, so why was I in such a funk? So much had changed. I could not possibly function at pre-event energy levels. Maybe life had taken a ninety-degree turn for a reason. Challenges often coax us into defining new missions for the life that lies ahead. Why wasn't I the least bit curious about what the new future would hold?

This was the opening act to a new beginning. The obsessed griever was ready to yield to the action-self. I had to let go. The past was the past, and there was no going back. Just short of the first anniversary of the ear event, I took the next big step on the road to acceptance, peace, and healing: *learning about hearing loss.*

The Power of Education

All of my life I have been a big believer in the power of education, because it gives us choices. At some point, it became clear that if I wanted to make sense of my case, I had to seriously study up. Vague questions had gotten vague answers and, over time, I had grown tired of living and breathing generic hearing loss. I wanted to know more—a lot more. With education comes information. Details fill in the knowledge blanks, and suddenly, the "big picture" comes together.

As the framework of information slowly built, it was easier to talk with my physicians and hearing specialists. Appointments became a lot more productive. The more I understood, the better I seemed to cope. Life with hearing loss, its consequences, and challenges began to make sense. In the end, I was able to accept reality and stopped asking "why?"

We all have different ways of dealing with adversity and pain. Throughout all of life's challenges and curve balls, I have always felt that learning about a given situation set me free in some way. In this case, it also turned out to be quite empowering and well worth the effort.

As time passed, I settled into my hearing loss, made peace with the ear phantom, and even found some humor in my off-and-on wobbliness or speech misunderstandings. I quit obsessing about my job. I let go of the fact that life was supposed to proceed the way it always had. I finally moved away from fixating on things that I could not change. I got peace within myself—the prerequisite toward a new beginning and future.

Attitude and Gratitude

Sir Winston Churchill is credited with the quote: "Attitude is a little thing that makes a big difference." I could not agree more, but in order to accept the truth of these words I had to rid myself of a lot of negative baggage along the way. With acceptance came an attitude softening that made moving forward so much easier. Over time, the "bad" ear has become the "injured" ear. I do not cuss at the ear phantom anymore—we simply live together as best we can. Instead of being seriously self-absorbed, I have turned much of my attention outward—towards others. I try to pay forward what I learned so that people can learn from me and with me. It is the major reason why I wrote this book.

While attitude is an important marker on the road to recovery, so is gratitude. At some point, a friend introduced the idea of keeping a Gratitude Journal, which forced me to focus on the positive rather than on repeating and reliving the negative. At first, I did not have much to report. Then, it dawned on me that under the circumstances, things could have been worse—a lot worse.

To this day, I am enormously grateful for the medical help that I received. I am grateful to those who never abandoned me as I inched forward, although I so often took them for granted and tested their patience and good will. Without the support of family, friends, and even total strangers, I would have had a much longer and more tedious row to hoe.

I am thankful to my husband for all his words of encouragement and for all the miles that he has hauled me in search of help for my ear, peace for my soul, and purpose for my life. I also thank him for his continued help, reassurance, and support while I wrote this book. Throughout the past few years, I have met many compassionate and giving people. I want to pass along what I learned to others who are in pain and confusion. I want to share the soothing words that were spoken to me.

All things considered, I got off easy. I often think of my personal heroes who are cancer survivors. Somewhere along the way, one of them said to me, so poignantly, that I would know when I was ready to stash away the past in favor of focusing on the future.

Now and then, I love to read quotes by famous people. Here is one from Hubert H. Humphrey, a fellow pharmacist, Minnesota senator, vice president, and overall caring and wise man: "Oh, my friend, it's not what they take away from you that counts. It's what you do with what you have left." How could anyone say it any better?

Nowadays, I spend less and less time peeking into the rearview mirror and spend more productive time developing strategies for my mission as a hearing-challenged person. I am aware of the losses that will always be part of the "new" me. I have healed more than I ever thought possible, and I am tremendously grateful for that. As a bonus, time has provided me with a cushion of homemade wisdom and humor to help on challenging days.

Chapter 41
Communication Challenges

Although I have made a lot of progress, there are some truths that cannot be denied. Depending on the circumstances, the mere acts of hearing and understanding become tiring work. Communication that used to be so easy has turned into yet another "job." It takes a lot of concentration and energy to follow a conversation. Talk about "listening fatigue!"

Hearing loss is often referred to as a *communication disorder*, and I have found this to be true. If hearing, listening, understanding, and responding are major communication features, then people with a hearing deficit are at a disadvantage on all counts. Social events and workplaces test our inner fortitude. In busy, noisy surroundings we might hear but fail to understand much of what is said because the pitches that make speech intelligible are blunted or lost. We hate questions. They are like "gotcha" tests because we cannot pretend anymore that we understand and let it all just pass. It is easy to see why this "communication disorder" quickly turns into a serious quality-of-life issue.

Another part of the communication job is to become proficient in electronics. Although they are now my helpers, I never knew much about sound systems, hearing aids, and assistive listening devices. It pays to learn about them and to be aware what is available on the market. I never read catalogs before, but now I do. After all, in order to be my best at the communication job, I need the correct tools.

Reconnecting with Society: to Bluff or to Disclose
Yes, I was in a funk over the events that beset me and climb-

ing out of the emotional quagmire was tough, but eventually, the time came to reconnect with society—but on different terms. The challenge was to position myself as a hard-of-hearing person within the hearing world. There were various options for handling this social reentry: I could bluff and deny my communication issues; or I could disclose them and stand my ground. I chose the latter.

Hearing loss is often called an *invisible* disability, but is it? It might be invisible because, on the outside, there is nothing obviously wrong with our perfect or even dainty ears. No one actually sees a dead or dying cochlea or a badly scarred ear drum. However, what does become noticeable to outsiders, is the effect that hearing loss has on communication behavior. In that sense, it is actually hard to hide. We become hesitant and act unsure of ourselves. We lean in and attempt to read lips. As those around us do notice such struggles, why would we pretend that everything is fine when it is not? Why would we show embarrassment when there is no need to do so?

Aware of the fact that they have hearing issues, there are those who willfully hide or deny their challenges and resort to bluffing and faking hearing. Considering the stigmas that surround hearing loss and how hard-of-hearing people are at times belittled and teased by coworkers or even family members and friends, this is easy to understand. The denial or bluffing mode, however, only feeds the stereotypical, obstructionist beliefs that hearing loss is a sign of decline or weakness. Bluffing can make a person look lost and disengaged, and often leads to conflicts and misunderstandings in both social and workplace settings.

Normalizing Communication Efforts

By now, my friends and most of my acquaintances know about my hearing status, that I am beset by tinnitus and often somewhat wobbly on my feet. The facts are the facts. I do not hide an ALD if one is needed, and I don't care if someone sees my hearing aid or finds out that I have one. In that sense, "honesty is the best policy" has turned out to be both liberating and empowering. Over the years, I have had many interesting conversations with people who wanted to learn about my ear event and who shared their own or a family member's challenges.

I decided early on that if I wanted to normalize my communication efforts, I had to disclose my hearing needs to those around me, depending on the situation, of course. I don't launch into unwelcome speeches, make major declarations in the grocery checkout line, or stand at the bus stop holding a banner. In order to do the communication job efficiently and with the least amount of trauma, I endeavor to reach out to others while hoping that they will accommodate me in return. Generally, social or professional contacts appreciate a statement such as, "I have a hearing loss. I might ask you to repeat whatever I don't catch, simply because everything that is said is important to me." Now, they no longer have to wonder or guess at my communication behavior.

I certainly cannot accuse others of being rude to me, of excluding me, and of mumbling if I never inform them that I have certain hearing limits and needs. I must also expect that I might have to kindly remind them—maybe by pointing to my ear—that they greatly help by speaking more slowly and by facing me. Most people try their best to be accommodating.

Communication Barriers and the Isolation Trap

One of the more insidious side effects of hearing loss is that it leads to social isolation, a most frustrating and stubborn affliction that often befalls those who wrestle with hearing issues. I got a taste of what it feels like and how much energy it takes to resist giving in to the negative impact that communication problems can have on life. Even now, the temptation is sometimes overwhelming to let myself drift toward Isolation Island rather than row against the treacherous currents that try to land me there. Communication hurdles are especially hard to overcome for those whose personalities tend naturally toward privacy or who lack a reliable support system.

What could make people so numb that they would withdraw from the social scene? Maybe they are just tired and have given up on fighting the daily battle of hearing loss. Maybe they cannot afford hearing aids and assistive devices. Maybe the "communication job" smothers and exhausts them. Maybe tinnitus, paired with hearing loss, robs them of their last remnants of resilience. Maybe they feel that people are critical and judgmental. Maybe they hide out because they do not want to be perceived as an embarrassment to others.

Not hearing, not understanding, misunderstanding, tiring easily, and having to rely on others to accommodate basic communication needs all erode self-confidence, self-esteem, and even hope. Avoidance of social contacts that are not absolutely necessary is the path of least resistance that many choose to take. However, what at first appears to be an easy solution can turn into a downhill slide that leads to social withdrawal and decreased quality of life.

As time goes on, it becomes easier and easier to find reasons for bowing out of meetings, family gatherings, or lunches with friends. ALDs and hearing aids do not generate excitement or interest anymore. Support group efforts maybe rejected as being unhelpful or unnecessary. Loneliness becomes a way of life, and for some, a gradual drift into substance abuse is a definite possibility. Social isolation should be a red flag to others that the person with hearing issues has deep-seated pain and that he or she needs their help more than ever. An invitation for a drive, for visiting a relative or friend, or for an outing to the park might be what it takes to break the cycle.

Need for Professional Help

That said, family and friends can be of great assistance, but they can only do so much. People with hearing loss must also understand that it is tough for those around them to see them suffer and turn into hermits. Once I realized that I was leading my family down that path, I did my best to ease and appreciate their efforts. Yet it is hard to admit to a shortcoming. It is hard to ask for help over and over and to still welcome it. It is hard to face into the wind day after day. It is hard to become dependent on others in so many ways. Eventually it is almost impossible for anyone to provide assistance or comfort and *professional help* becomes the next step.

Professional help, however, must come from counselors who are experienced in working with people whose hearing loss holds them hostage. They must be familiar with the diverse aspects of the condition and how it impacts people's lives. Unfortunately, many report that their therapists have little or no understanding for their challenges. They might not even know the basic rules for communicating with their clients. Therefore, if professional advice is required, we must always ask about the clinician's expertise with hearing loss. For deaf people, it is a huge advantage if the therapist knows sign language.

I developed great respect for hearing-loss savvy professionals when a specialized psychologist gave a few talks to our support group. No question or comment stomped or surprised her. She was compassionate with loads of practical tips and advice, but she also had that little spark of toughness that people who are stuck in the isolation bog need in order to work themselves out. She introduced us to the notion of *Radical Acceptance*. At some point, one has to let go and quit the self-torture with questions for which there may be no or few answers. It simply is what it is. She basically reinforced what our daughter had already tried to tell me. This most insightful moment became a turning point on my hearing loss recovery journey.

Yes, there is help. Luckily, I had a supportive family and caring friends who kept me from becoming shipwrecked on infamous Isolation Island—a notable Gratitude Journal entry.

Chapter 42
Gateways to the World of Hearing Loss: Associations, Organizations, Support Groups

When I first lost my hearing and was tortured by tinnitus, my husband took me to a meeting of the local chapter of the Hearing Loss Association of America (HLAA). I think that he did so out of sheer desperation. It is hard to live with someone who is in constant upheaval, who talks about things that do not make much sense, and who obviously needs some coping skills. He thought that I should meet people who could understand what and how I felt. I am forever grateful to him for nudging me into the world of hearing loss, a threshold that I had become ready to cross.

The HLAA mission statement is to "open the world of communication to people with hearing loss by providing information, education, support and advocacy." Although the need for information and support first took me there, I have since become quite active in the area of advocacy.

Within the hearing loss community, we must make it our goal to work seriously on our self-confidence and self-worth. A good first step is to acknowledge the facts. The truth is that as long as so many of us dwell on denying, hiding, or ignoring the obvious, we remain stuck in our current position: under-recognized, under-represented, stereotyped into oblivion, and seriously misunderstood.

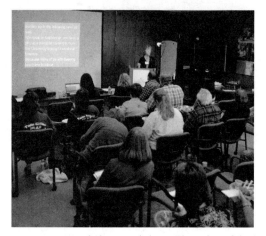

In support groups people learn and share. The value of the human connection is priceless. *photo: R.Hammond*

At our first meeting there were adults from all walks of life and from all age groups. Some people had a gradual hearing decline, while others were born with hearing loss. Most had hearing aids. Some were brought back, at least partially, to the hearing world, thanks to a cochlear implant. Some had Ménière's Disease. Some had tinnitus, and others did not. Besides my husband, other fully hearing people had accompanied a friend or a family member to the meeting, simply because they wanted to understand the challenges of hearing-related disorders better. They came to find ways to help and support their loved ones. How uplifting is that?

I quickly learned that I was a total greenhorn and that my lot was a breeze compared to the lifetime of ear quandaries that some of my new brethren endured. In many ways it was a humbling experience. Yet the common bond that we shared made it amazingly easy to talk about rather personal things to a room full of strangers.

Over the years we have had scores of informative presentations by top-notch professionals who graciously and willingly shared their expertise with regard to hearing and tinnitus issues. We have been instructed by a truly awesome cast of audiologists, doctors, researchers from the hearing aid and assistive listening device industries, government agency representatives, law enforcement agents, politicians, personal safety experts, lawyers specializing in disability issues, psychotherapists, and our own member specialists. I have truly never left a meeting without having gotten new information.

Most of all, the "ear meetings" put me in contact with some outstanding and brave people whom I otherwise would not have had the honor and privilege to meet. They breathed new optimism into me by demonstrating that life with hearing loss and tinnitus is indeed manageable. Subsequently, I became vice president and then president of our HLAA chapter, which offered a special opportunity to give back to the people who welcomed me and encouraged me when I was a bit of a mess.

I also attend meetings sponsored by the International Hearing Foundation (IHF). This group focuses mostly on Ménière's Disease and on the ear phantom, tinnitus. In these monthly gatherings, we mostly share and talk. Sometimes we have a speaker. The relaxed and safe environment of acceptance and fellowship is soothing to the mind and soul.

Although most towns do not have official association chapters or "live" support groups, there are online sites that connect people who are hard of hearing. Try the Hearing Loss Association of America (HLAA) at http://www.hearingloss.org/content/message-boardschat-rooms

For young adults: http://www.hearingloss.org/content/young-adults-0

A Special Note on Support Groups

The notion of "support group" is often misunderstood by the public. Support groups, live or in cyberspace, are *not* substitutes for appropriate medical care. Live meetings are facilitated social gatherings where people with similar challenges or adversities find a safe haven among their own. Those who attend can speak without having to be afraid that they upset family, friends, or their boss. It simply feels comforting to know that we are not alone and that there are people out there who understand our situation.

Certainly, attendees share their feelings and experiences, but the calling of a support group is *not* to dispense medical advice, give doctor and practitioner referrals, or second-guess treatment plans. Unfortunately, distressed newcomers or those who feel let down by the medical/audiology systems don't always understand this. All too often they expect immediate solutions for their unresolved issues. Dealing with hearing challenges, however, is a journey of adjustment and discovery, not a whirlwind search for ready-made answers.

Although they might not be helpful for all, support groups have been tremendously important in my new life. They gave me refuge when I was distraught, and I hope that I can pass along to others the message of encouragement that I received. It's simply a matter of gratitude.

Chapter 43
Future Outlook:
Research, Education, Prevention

According to Johns Hopkins Medicine, by now one in five Americans, age *twelve* and over, has hearing loss significant enough to make communication difficult. Statistics are numbers that help us study trends, and the numbers for hearing loss are "trending upward," not only among our aging population but, more alarmingly, among younger people. As most cases of tinnitus are linked to hearing loss, we can conclude that tinnitus, too, is on the rise. The financial burden for diagnosing and treating hearing loss and its consequences will weigh heavily on future family and government health care budgets.

As we have seen, there currently is no cure for sensorineural hearing loss or tinnitus, but revolutionary treatments for both conditions will be in the future. Cochlear hair cell regeneration by means of stem cell therapy or gene therapy or topical drugs is a field of intense research, and progress is being slowly made. For scientists, the major challenges are how to keep regenerated cells alive and how to make them fully functional so that they will be able to carry out the sound-sensing and tuning duties of their dead forerunners.

I take great solace in the fact that in medicine revolutionary advances have often been made almost overnight. While I hold great hope for positive outcomes, help in the form of new cochlear cells still lies in the somewhat distant future. Until then, we must take stock of the hearing realities that impact us in the now. Electronics will obviously play an ever-increasing role in day-to-day communications, but they will not be able to compensate for the human, social, and quality-of-life issues that hearing loss can bestow on the individual.

Saving Ears—Two at a Time!

Regardless of research and technology, it makes sense that the smartest strategies are still patient education as well as prevention and management of risk factors. As hearing loss is considered a symptom of an underlying condition, it must never be ignored, and getting a medical opinion is of great importance. Maybe it is not just aging! Instead, people take between five and ten years before they act on their symptoms, thereby possibly wasting valuable time. Most of all, we must protect the ears from excessive noise, the single most preventable cause of hearing damage. Turning down the volume in our overly loud lives is a good start.

Over time, I have become the sworn enemy of ear-damaging sound. Noise-induced hearing loss (NIHL) is rampant especially among younger people whose ears age way before their time. Then, according to the Occupational Safety and Health Administration (OSHA), "every year, approximately thirty million people in the United States are occupationally exposed to hazardous noise." That said, every-day-life is getting louder too. The bottom line is that, as a society, we must become ear-smart and hearing-wise to noise.

I have worked for a number of years on noise-related hearing issues. The goal is to raise awareness and to educate the public for the purpose of preventing NIHL. Many people do not realize that the devastation that they inflict on their ears will have dire quality-of-life consequences.

Throughout my years in health care, I have always been a big believer in Benjamin Franklin's wise words that "an ounce of prevention is worth a pound of cure." Now that hearing loss has surfaced as my new life mission, I stick to this conviction. As prevention has its roots in education, I know that this is the road that I will continue to travel, simply because I believe that knowledge that is not shared is worthless. It is not "power," as we like to say. It becomes powerful when others become the wiser.

Early on, I read a quote by Dr. Martin Luther King Jr. that both inspired and awed me. It felt like he issued a personal dare to me and to others with hearing problems: "Our lives begin to end the day we become silent about things that matter." With hearing loss, there is so much that matters—or should matter—to us and to society as a whole that silence is simply not an option, not now and not in the future. For me this means that I will continue my efforts according to my motto: *Saving Ears—Two at a Time!*

PART EIGHT
APPENDIX

The following checklists are provided to help prepare for visits with the professionals. My experience taught me that ear- and hearing-related problems of any kind must be checked out medically. During the various test routines and doctor visits I often wondered why everybody asked the same things over and over. Then I determined that every specialist looked at the problem from a different angle or point of view. The more detail I could provide, the better it was. I put some checklists together in order to get our thought process started as we *prepare for appointments* with various hearing professionals. These lists do not cover all possible issues and concerns by any means. Questions and suggestions may overlap but I hope that they are a good beginning for proceeding in the right direction.

APPENDIX

Checklists

1 **Preparing for a Primary Care Physician Appointment Regarding Hearing Loss**
2 **Preparing for Hearing Tests**
3 **Preparing for an Ear Specialist Appointment**
4 **Selecting a Hearing Aid Vendor**
5 **Buying a Hearing Aid**
6 **Buying a Hearing Aid: The T-coil**
7 **Preparing for a Doctor Appointment Regarding Tinnitus**
8 **Preparing for an Audiologist Appointment Regarding Tinnitus Treatment**
9 **Selected Information Websites (in alphabetical order)**

Checklist 1

Preparing for a Primary Care Physician Appointment Regarding Hearing Loss

Any hearing loss should be evaluated medically. A *concise history* of the condition itself and of the patient's health and family histories can provide important information in the search for a possible underlying cause. Due to insurance constraints, many patients start with their primary physician, who will then refer them to a *specialist*. The waiting periods to see a specialist can be lengthy. How can your doctor help speed up the process?

NOTE: A **sudden** persistent hearing loss that happened over no more than three days is a medical ***emergency***. Seek medical help at once.

1. Write all your information, hunches, and questions down.
2. Think of any contributing factors. Loud noise exposures? Stress? New medication(s)? Injuries? Frequent colds? Recurring sinus or ear infections? Other_____
3. Do you have any other symptoms: headaches, tinnitus, sinus trouble, dizziness, ear pain or fullness?
4. Is one ear affected or are both ears involved?
5. Do hearing issues run in the family? Explain.
6. *When* did you become aware that your hearing has de creased?
7. *How* did you become aware of the loss? Somebody told you so?
8. When are you bothered the most? At home? At work? When socializing?
9. Think about the noise levels at work and at home.

How do you rate your hearing now on a scale from 1 to 10? (10 = perfect)

10. What would you have rated your hearing before the loss?
11. What other doctors do you see currently for regular care?
    Condition(s)?
12. Take **all** medications—prescription and non-prescription
    —vitamins and supplements to the doctor for review.

Checklist 2

Preparing for Hearing Tests

Note: The doctor, preferably a specialist, will ask that diagnostic hearing tests be done by an *audiologist before* the actual appointment. I had my ears tested by audiologists affiliated with the ENT clinic. Looking back, this eliminated the commercial and sales bias. The focus was on "diagnosis" where it should have been. If tests are done elsewhere, be sure that the audiologist's name and contact information figure on the test record in case of questions. Some of the following questions are already covered in Checklist #1. Here are a few extra suggestions in order to get the most out of the hearing test visit.

1. Be prepared to give a full account of your hearing, health, and family histories.
2. How many steps does the set of hearing tests involve?
3. What part of the ear and hearing does each step test?
4. Have each step of the procedure explained so that you know what to expect.
5. Know what your role is for each phase of the testing process.
6. Ask for an explanation of any technical expressions.
7. If you have *tinnitus*, tell the audiologist. The test signal will be adjusted so that it can be distinguished from the sounds of tinnitus.
8. The audiologist must inspect the ears as the first step of the tests.
9. For reliable results, wax build-ups must be removed *before* the tests.
10. During the test, speak up or signal if you are uncomfortable. The tester can see and hear you.
11. After the test ask to see the tracings. What do they reveal? (Answering such questions is often left to the doctor.)
12. Ask for a paper copy of the audiogram for your file. This will help if and when you are released to check on hearing aids.

APPENDIX

Checklist 3
Preparing for an Ear Specialist Appointment
Write down all questions and concerns. Complete Checklist #1. Bring the copy of the audiogram. Depending on the case, be ready for additional tests to be ordered or for referrals to other specialists.

1. According to the hearing tests and doctor's findings, what type of hearing loss do you have?
2. What might have caused the loss? Can anything be treated or fixed?
3. Which frequencies are affected?
4. How serious is the loss?
5. What is the diagnosis?
6. What does that mean for you professionally, socially, etc.?
7. Might a hearing aid be helpful?
8. Discuss other symptoms such as tinnitus or dizziness. What might they be due to? Can they be treated?
9. What is your major concern? Job? Family? Marriage? Going deaf altogether?
10. Will you need more tests? Which ones?
11. What kind of helpful answers will the extra tests provide?
12. Must you consult additional specialists? Check on your *insurance coverage*. Are *referrals* needed before proceeding?
13. Are the strategies for managing your condition acceptable? Why not?
14. If *medications* are prescribed review them in detail with the doctor as to purpose and side effects
15. Is there a time limit on the medication treatment regimes?
16. When must you contact the doctor ASAP regarding your medications?
17. If you are released to check on a hearing aid, be sure to get a *medical release form* to give to the vendor.

Checklist 4

Selecting a Hearing Aid Vendor

Note: Buying a hearing aid is based on a *trust relationship* between client and vendor. When checking out a store or clinic, get to know the practitioner. Ask questions and screen for obvious red flags.

1. Does the store/clinic sell all types of hearing aids?
2. Is the store an *outlet* that deals only with the wares of a *specific* manufacturer?
3. What does that mean for you? Limitations and benefits?
4. Does the vendor give information on the benefits of ALDs?
5. Check out vendor professional credentials. Audiologist? HID? Other?
6. Is the vendor accredited to practice by the state?
7. Are valid state license or certification papers displayed in the office?
8. Although it is not necessary, is the specialist board certified?
9. How long has the specialist been active in *direct* customer service?
10. Does the specialist ask up front for a medical release statement as required?
11. Does the vendor inform you of the requirement of a medical check?
12. Does the vendor encourage the signing of a medical consult waiver?
13. Does the specialist try to understand your specific needs and case?
14. Is the interview all about the sale and little about your hearing needs?
15. Does the specialist inform you of the need for follow-up adjustment visits?
16. Will your hearing be retested? Why or why not?

17. Is there a charge for the test, even if you decide not to buy at this time?
18. Does the specialist discuss the store trial policy?
19. Will the days spent waiting for adjustments be added to the trial period?
20. Does the vendor agree to give any verbal agreements in writing?
21. Will you be given time to review all contract, sales and warranty details?
22. Remember that patient/practitioner compatibility is important for best results.
23. Will you be able to schedule with the *same* specialist in the future?
24. What is the practitioner's score on your trust-o-meter? High? Iffy? No go?

Checklist 5
Buying a Hearing Aid
After working through checklist #4 and finding a compatible hearing specialist, the search for an instrument begins. Mention any issues like tinnitus, hyperacusis, and problems with infections or ear wax up front. Bring any audiograms for review and for comparison in case that the ears are retested.

1. Does the specialist check the outer ears for problems? Inquire about the findings.
2. If the hearing is tested, have each step explained.
3. Ask to have the final test tracings explained.
4. Do the specialist's statements agree with your doctor's account?
5. How do the test results influence the instrument choice?
6. If only one ear is involved, make sure that the *correct one* is fitted!
7. Why is the suggested device the most appropriate one? Ask for details.
8. Do you need all the described features or do they only add to the costs? (wireless capabilities, Bluetooth, number of channels, etc.)
9. Does the specialist only talk about the very positive aspects of the aid?
10. What are the instrument's limitations or downsides?
11. Sticker shock? Is there an equally effective, less pricey choice?
12. Comparison shop.
13. Are *real-ear* measures done during the setting/programming phase?
14. Do any extras come with the device? How much do they cost?
15. Is there a limit on the number of adjustment visits during the trial period?
16. How much is the down-payment?

17. How much will be refunded in case that the device is returned?
18. How long is the manufacturer warranty? What is covered?
19. Do you need additional insurance coverage? Does it cover what the manufacturer's warranty does not cover?
20. Review all paperwork and *do read* the fine print *before* signing any agreement.

Checklist 6
Buying a Hearing Aid: The T-coil

1. Depending on the instrument it might not apply, but ask about a T-coil option.
2. Would a T-coil benefit you? Why not?
3. Is the T-coil already installed in the aid?
4. *If yes*, does the instrument price include the coil price?
5. Does it cost extra to activate/program the coil?
6. If the coil is activated, are real-ear measurements done?
7. If the device does *not* have a t-coil, can one be installed? Why not?
8. What is the cost for adding a coil?
9. Is it covered by warranty? Get details.
10. How is it maintained?
11. With what types of phones and other ALDs is the T-coil compatible?
12. Get instructions for optimal benefit and use.

APPENDIX

Checklist 7
Preparing for a Doctor's Appointment Regarding Tinnitus
Tinnitus is often a consequence of hearing loss, but not always. Tinnitus should be medically evaluated since it can be a symptom of some other underlying condition. It is important to find a doctor who has an *interest in the tinnitus patient*. Be prepared to give a detailed account and to submit to some medical and hearing tests. Take *all* medications, herbal products, supplements, etc. to the appointment.

1. When did the ear/head noises start?
2. What does the tinnitus sound like? Buzzing? Hissing? Pulsing? Swishing?
3. Is it continuous or off-and-on?
4. If it is intermittent, what seems to bring it on?
5. Are the noises related to head, neck, jaw, or eye movements?
6. Are you depressed, stressed, or anxious?
7. Think of possible causes: new medication(s), noise exposure, sinus issues, allergies, etc.
8. On a scale from 1 to 10, how loud is the tinnitus? (10 being loudest)
9. What makes it worse?
10. What seems to soothe it?
11. Does it interfere with sleeping?
12. How does it affect your life?
13. Are any aggravating factors treatable?
14. If tests are ordered, find out what they are for, and what they will disclose,
15. If medications are ordered, find out exactly what they are,
16. Ask how the medication will help and what you can expect,
17. Ask about side effects and possible treatment time limitations,
18. Review the exact dosing instructions with the physician; what does "as needed" mean?

19. When must you return for a follow-up visit?
20. Ask about other treatment options: masking, sound therapy, etc.
21. Ask for a written referral to a special tinnitus clinic for evaluation, if needed.

APPENDIX

Checklist 8
Preparing for an Audiologist's Appointment Regarding Tinnitus Treatment

1. Be prepared to give an account of your tinnitus:
   When did it start? What does it sound like? Is it constant or intermittent? How does it affect your life?
2. Have you seen a medical doctor about the noises? Name & specialty?
3. What was his/her opinion or diagnosis?
4. What has already been tried?
5. Inquire about the different treatments, such as masking options: TRT, Neuromonics, Ultrasound, etc.
6. If maskers are to be used, clarify costs, trial time, refunds, instrument warranty, payment schedules
7. Might the use of masking noises/music (CDs, programmed MP3 player) be just as effective?
8. If TRT or Neuromonics are to be tried, inquire about the audiologist's training certification in these techniques.
9. How many patients has the clinic treated successfully?
10. Share your expectations as far as therapy results are concerned
11. Why is one treatment chosen over the other?
12. Clarify the details of the therapy such as timelines, costs, and refunds.
13. Clarify the directive counseling issue: how many sessions will you have? How will the counseling be administered? Face-to-face? By phone? By email?
14. Will you be working with the same therapist for the duration of the treatment?
15. Can you change in case of problems or personality issues?
16. Will any post-treatment follow-up visits be included in the package?

Checklist 9

Selection of Information Websites (in alphabetical order)
- Alexander Graham Bell Association for the Deaf and Hard of Hearing
www.agbell.org
- American Association of the Deaf-Blind (AADB)
www.aadb.org
- American Speech-Language-Hearing Association (ASHA)
www.asha.org
- American Tinnitus Association National Headquarters (ATA)
www.ata.org
- Comprehensive Site for Hyperacusis Information
www.hyperacusis.org
- Hearing Loss Association of America (HLAA)
www.hearingloss.org
- Hyperacusis Network
http://www.hyperacusis.net
- Ménière's Disease Information Center (MDIC)
www.menieresinfo.com
- National Association of the Deaf (NAD)
www.nad.org
- National Dizzy and Balance Center (NDBC)
www.stopdizziness.com
- National Institute on Deafness and Other Communication Disorders (NIDCD)
www.nidcd.nih.gov
- National Institute for Occupational Safety and Health (NIOSH)
www.cdc.gov/niosh
- Occupational Safety and Health Administration (OSHA)
www.osha.gov
- Vestibular Disorders Association (VEDA)
www.vestibular.org

REFERENCES ARRANGED
BY CHAPTER

Chapter 3 - D-DAY and Beyond

Bauman, Neil. "Sudden Sensorineural Hearing Loss (SSHL*)*." *Center for Hearing Loss Help*. June 2007. <http://www.hearinglosshelp.com/articles/suddenhearingloss>

Kaltenbach, James. "A Breakthrough in Hair Cell Regeneration." *Tinnitus Today* June 2003: 12-13. Print.

Chapter 4 - In Search of Medical Help

Boston, Mark E., Strasnick, Barry, and Steinberg, Amalia R. "Inner Ear, Labyrinthitis." *eMedicine Neurology*. January 2010. <http://emedicine.medscape.com/article/inner-ear/labyrinthitis>

Hain, Timothy C. "Benign Paroxysmal Positional Vertigo." *Dizziness-and-balance.com*. July 2009. <http://www.dizziness-and-balance.com/disorders/bppv>

Hain, Timothy C. "Vestibular Neuritis and Labyrinthitis." *Dizziness-and-balance.com*. September 2009. <http://www.dizziness-and-balance.com/disorders/unilat/vneurit.html>

Mayo Clinic Staff. "Benign paroxysmal positional vertigo (BPPV)." *MayoClinic.com*. May 2008. <http://www.mayoclinic.com/health/bppv>

REFERENCES ARRANGED BY CHAPTER

Chapter 11 - Road Map for the Journey

American Speech-Language-Hearing Association. "How Hearing and Balance Work." June 2009. <http://www.asha.org/public/hearing/anatomy>

Bruns, Alan D., Ruckenstein, Michael J, and Bedrosian, Jeffrey. "Middle Ear Function." *eMedicine Otolaryngology and Facial Plastic Surgery.* July 2008. <http://emedicine.medscape.com/article/874456-overview>

Jacob, Stanley W. and Francone, Clarice A. "Auditory Sense." *Structure and Function in Man.* Third Edition. Chapter 9:295-300. Pennsylvania: W.B. Saunders Company, 1974. Print.

Kaltenbach, James. "A Breakthrough in Hair Cell Regeneration." *Tinnitus Today.* June 2003: 12-13. Print

Marieb, Elaine N., Mallatt, Jon, and Wilhelm, Patricia B. "The Ear: Hearing and Equilibrium." *Human Anatomy.* Fourth Edition. Chapter 16: 467-479. California: Pearson Benjamin Cummings, 2005. Print.

Salt, Alec N. "A Pictorial Guide to the Cochlear Fluids." *Cochlear Fluids Research Laboratory.* Washington University, St. Louis. N.d. Retrieved March 2010. <http://oto2.wustl.edu/cochlea/intro1.html>

Chapter 12 - Audiology and Hearing Tests

American Speech-Language-Hearing Association. "Hearing Screening and Testing: Types of Tests used to Evaluate Hearing in Children and Adults." N.d. Retrieved July 2009. <http://www.asha.org/public/hearing/Hearing-Testing>

Bruns, Alan D., Ruckenstein, Michael J., and Bedrosian, Jeffrey. "Middle Ear Function: Assessment of Middle Ear Function." *eMedicine Otolaryngology and Facial Plastic Surgery.* July 2008. <http://emedicine.medscape.com/article/874456-overview>

Campbell, Kathleen C M and Mullen, Ginger. "Impedance Audiometry." *eMedicine Clinical Procedures.* December 2009. <http://emedicine.medscape.com/article/1831254-overview>

Hain, Timothy C. "Hearing Testing." *Dizziness-and-balance.com.* October 2009. <http://www.dizziness-and-balance.com/testing/hearing-test>

Hain, Timothy C. "OAE Testing (Otoacoustic Emissions)." *Dizziness-and-balance.com.* Jan 2011. <www.dizziness-and-balance.com/testing/hearing/OAE.htm>

Hain, Timothy C. "Brainstem Auditory Evoked Responses (BAER or ABR)." *Dizziness-and-balance.com.* April 2010. <http://www.dizziness-and-balance.com/testing/hearing/baer.htm>

Kutz, Joe W. Jr., Mullen, Ginger, and Campbell, Kathleen C M. "Audiology, Pure-Tone Testing." *eMedicine Otolaryngology and Facial Plastic Surgery.* June 2008. <http://www.emedicine.com/ent/TOPIC311.HTMl>

Ruben, Robert J.,ed. " Hearing loss: Introduction." *The Merck*

Manuals Online Medical Library. September 2009. <http://www.merckmanuals.com/professional/sec08/ch085/ch085a. html>

Chapter 13 - The Elements of an Audiogram

Bauman, Neil. "Hearing Loss - Decibels or Percent?"(decibel as ratio). *Center for Hearing Loss Help.* February 2003. <http://www.hearinglosshelp.com/articles/decibelsvspercent.html>

Brown, Steven. "General Acoustics." *Listen Hear Sound Projects.* N.d. Retrieved July 2008. <http://www.listenhear.co.uk/general-acoustics.html>

Bruns, Alan D., Ruckenstein, Michael J., and Bedrosian, Jeffrey. "Middle Ear Function: What is sound?" *eMedicine Otolaryngology and Facial Plastic Surgery*; July 2008. <http://emedicine.medscape.com/article/874456-overview>

CDC – NIOSH. "Noise and Hearing Loss Prevention. Noise Meter." May 2010. <www.cdc.gov/niosh/topics/noise/noisemeter-flash.html>

Dangerous Decibels. "Hearing Loss. How loud is too loud?" N.d. Retrieved July 2008. <http://www.dangerousdecibels.org/how-loud-is-too-loud>

Hain, Timothy C. "Audiometry." *Dizziness-and-balance.com.* June 2009. <http://www.dizziness-and-balance.com/testing/hearing/audiogram. html>

Kutz, Joe Walter, Mullen, Ginger, and Campbell, Kathleen CM. "Audiology, Pure-tone Testing. Types of Hearing Loss." *eMedicine Otolaryngology and Facial and Plastic Surgery.* June 2008.
<http://emedicine.com/ent/topic311.HTM>

PBS: The American Experience. "More about Bell. A Family Affair." N.d. Retrieved May 2010.
<http://pbs.org/wgbh/amex/telephone/peopleevents/mabell.html>

Ruben, Robert J.,ed. "Hearing loss: Testing". *The Merck Manuals Online Medical Library.* September 2009.
<http://www.merckmanuals.com/professional/sec08/ch085/ch085a.html>

SPARKMUSEUM. "The Discovery of Radio Waves 1888. Heinrich Rudolf Hertz." N.d. Retrieved May 2010.
<http://www.sparkmuseum.com/BOOK-HERTZ>

Chapter 14 - Quantifying a Hearing Loss

American Speech-Language-Hearing Association. "Degree of Hearing loss." N.d. Retrieved April 2009.
<http://www.asha.org/Degree-of-Hearing-Loss>

Bauman, Neil. "Hearing Loss: Decibels or Percent? Classifying Our Hearing Loss." *Center for Hearing Loss Help.* February 2003.
<http://www.hearinglosshelp.com/articles/decibelsvspercent>

Bauman, Neil. "How Much Are You Worth as a Hard of Hearing Person?"(Percent Disability). *Center for Hearing Loss Help.*

September 2001.
<http://www.hearinglosshelp.com/articles/hohworth>

Dobie, Robert A. "Percentage of Hearing Loss." (Calculations in hearing loss compensation). *Audiology Online Ask the Expert.* 6 July 2001.
<http://www.audiologyonline.com/askexpert/percentage-of-hearing-loss>

Kutz, Joe Walter, Mullen, Ginger, and Campbell, Kathleen C M. Audiology, Pure-tone Testing. "Pure-tone average (PTA)." *eMedicine Otolaryngology and Facial and Plastic Surgery.* June 2008.
<http://emedicine.com/ent/topic311.HTM>

Chapter 15 - The Many Causes of Hearing Loss

American Academy of Otolaryngology-Head and Neck Surgery. "Fact Sheet: What You Should Know About Otosclerosis." N.d. Retrieved April 2010.
<http://entnet.org/HealthInformation/otosclerosis.cfm>

Hain, Timothy C. "Autoimmune Inner Ear Disease (A.I.E.D)." *Dizziness-and-balance.com.* November 2010.
<http://www.dizziness-and-balance.com/disorders/autoimmune/aied>

Hain, Timothy C. "OTOSYPHILIS."*Dizziness-and-balance.com.* June 2009.
<http://www.dizziness-and-balance.com/otosyphilis>

National Institute on Deafness and Other Communication Disorders. "Quick Statistics." June 2010. <http://www.nidcd.nih.gov/health/statistics/quick.htm>

Neurotology Research Center, Metropolitan Ear Group, Inc. Bethesda, MD. "Tumors: Cholesteatoma." N.d. Retrieved April 2010. <http://www.earsite.com/cholesteatoma>

Maryland, University of, Medical Center. "Acoustic Neuroma/ Vestibular Schwannoma." N.d. Retrieved March 2010. <http://www.umm.edu/otolaryngology/acoustic-neuromas.html>

Mathur, Neeraj N. "Inner Ear, Autoimmune Disease." *eMedicine Otolaryngology and Facial Plastic Surgery.* October 2009. <http://emedicine.medscape.com/article/857511-overview>

MedlinePlus Medical Encyclopedia. "Otosclerosis." August 2010. <http://www.nlm.nih.gov/medlineplus/ency/article/001036.html>

Roland, Peter S. "Cholesteatoma." *eMedicine Otolaryngology and Facial Plastic Surgery.* June 2009. <http://emedicine.medscape.com/article/860080-overview>

Vestibular Disorder Association (VEDA). "Autoimmune Inner Ear Disease (AIED)." August 2010. <http://www.vestibular.org/vestibular-disorders/autoimmunity>

WebMD. "Hearing Loss: Cause." August 2009. <http://www.webmd.com/a-to-z-guides/hearing-loss-cause>

REFERENCES ARRANGED BY CHAPTER

Chapter 16 - Noise-Induced Hearing Loss (NIHL)

Acoustical Society of America (ASA). "Noise-induced hidden hearing loss mechanism discovered." *ScienceDaily* 7 May 2014. <www.sciencedaily.com/releases/2014/05/140507142804.htm>

Centers for Disease Control (CDC). Healthy Youth! "Noise-Induced Hearing Loss." March 2010. <http://www.cdc.gov/healthyyouth/noise>

Cooper Safety Supply. "Noise Reduction Ratings Explained." N.d. Retrieved October 2010. <http://www.coopersafety.com/NoiseReduction.aspx>

Dancer, Jess. "Antioxidants: An Antidote for Noise-Induced Hearing Loss?" *Hearing Loss Web. N.d. Retrieved.* May 2010. <http://www.hearinglossweb.com/Medical/cures/drug/jess.htm>

Dangerous Decibels. "Hearing Loss. How loud is too loud?" July 2008. <http:// www.dangerousdecibels.org/how-loud-is-too-loud>

Finz, Stacy. "The Din of Dining." *The Chronicle.* June 4, 2008. <http://www.sfgate.com/din-of-dining>

Francis, R. Patrick. "Your brain may be playing tricks with your hearing!" *Francis Audiology Associates.* January 2007. <http://www.francisaudiology.com/yourbrainmaybeplayingtrick-swithyourhearing.html>

Michigan, University of. Press Release: "Nutrients May Prevent Noise-Induced Hearing Loss." *Hearing Loss Web*. March 2007. <http://www.hearinglossweb.com/Medical/Causes/nihl/prtct/nutr.>

National Institute on Deafness and Other Communication Disorders (NIDCD). "Noise-Induced Hearing Loss." October 2008. <http://www.nidcd.nih.gov/health/hearing/noise.asp>

Neitzel, Rick. "NIOSH and OSHA Permissible Noise Exposure Limits." *Audiology Online Ask the Expert*. 29 September 2008. <http://www.audiologyonline.com/askexpert/permissible-noise>

Occupational Safety and Health Administration (OSHA). "What Constitutes an Effective Hearing Conservation Program?" N.d. Retrieved July 2008.
<http://www.osha.gov/dts/osta/otm/noise/hcp/sectionIV.html>

Thelen, Thom. "Perception Vs. Reality: What Our Ears Hear." *Acoustics By Design*. 12 December 2008.
<http://www.acousticsbydesign.com/acoustics-blog/perception-vs-reality.html>

World Health Organization (WHO): "1.1 Billion People at Risk of Hearing Loss." February 2015.
<http://www.who.int/mediacentre/news/releases/2015/ear-care/en/>

Chapter 17 - Ototoxic Substances

Bauman, Neil G. *Ototoxic Drugs Exposed*. Third Edition. Pennsylvania:Integrity First Publications, 2010. Print

REFERENCES ARRANGED BY CHAPTER

Curhan, Sharon G., Eavey, Roland, Shargorodsky, Joseph, Curhan, Gary C. "Analgesic Use and the Risk of Hearing Loss in Men." *The American Journal of Medicine.* March 2010.
<http://www.amjmed.com/article/S0002-9343(09)00795-5/abstract>

Drugwatch.com. "Drug Side Effects: Tinnitus." April 2011.
<http://www.drugwatch.com/side-effects>

FDA: Postmarket Drug Safety Information. "Possible Sudden Hearing Loss. Questions and Answers aboutViagra, Levitra, Cialis, and Revatio." October 2007.
<http://www.fda.gov/drugs/hearing-loss/106525>

Hain, Timothy C. "Ototoxic Medications." Otoneurology Education Index. N.d. Retrieved March 2009.
<http://www.tchain.com/otoneurology/disorders/ototoxins.html>

Maddox, P.T, Saunders, J., Chandrasekhar, S.S. Abstract: "Sudden Hearing Loss from PDE-5 Inhibitors. A Possible Cellular Stress Etiology." August 2009. *PubMed.gov.*
<http://www.ncbi.nlm.nih.gov/pubmed/19507217>

Pray W. Steven and Pray Joshua, J. "Ototoxic Medications." *US Pharmacist.* October 2005.24,26,28,30. Print.

Vestibular Disorder Association (VEDA). "Ototoxicity." February 2010.
<http://www.vestibular.org/ototoxicity>

Chapter 18 - The MRI

Brown, Nancy Marie. "Improving MRI." *Research/Penn State.* 16(2) June 1995.
<http://www.rps.psu.edu/jun95/mri.html>

Katsunuma, A., Takamori H., Sakakura, Y., Hamamura, Y., Ogo, Y., Katayama, R. Abstract: "Quiet MRI with Novel Acoustic Noise Reduction." January 2002. *PubMed.gov.*
<http://www.ncbi.nlm.nih.gov/pubmed/11755088>

National Research Council Canada. "Gradient Free MRI (silent)." February 2010.
<http://www.nrc-cnrc.gc.ca/eng/gradient-free-mri.html>

Sanders, Barbara T. "MRIs; The Noise Inside the Tube." *Tinnitus Today.* March 2006. 4-5. Print.

WebMD. "Magnetic Resonance Imaging (MRI)."June 2009.
<http://webmd.com/a-to-z-guides/magnetic-resonance-imaging-mri>

Chapter 19 - Tumors

Hoag Gamma Knife Center. "What is Gamma Knife?" N.d. Retrieved August 2008.
<http://hoaghospital.org/WhatisGammaKnife>

Kutz, Joe Walter, Roland, Peter S. and Isaacson, Brandon. "Skull Base, Acoustic Neuroma (Vestibular Schwannoma)." *eMedicine Otolaryngology and Facial Plastic Surgery.* September 2009.
<http://emedicine.medscape.com/article/882876-overview>

Maryland, University of, Medical Center. "Acoustic Neuroma/ Vestibular Schwannoma." N.d. Retrieved March 2010. <http://www.umm.edu/otolaryngology/acoustic-neuromas.html>

National Institute on Deafness and Other Communication Disorders. "Vestibular Schwannoma (Acoustic Neuroma) and Neurofibromatosis." February 2004. <http://www.nidcd.nih.gov/health/acoustic-neuroma.asp>

Chapter 20 - Equilibrium and Balance: Ears, Eyes, and Body Sensors

American Speech-Language-Hearing Association. "How Our Balance System Works." N.d. Retrieved July 2008. <http://www.asha.org/How-Our-Balance-System-Works>

Hain, Timothy C. "Benign Paroxysmal Positional Vertigo." *Dizziness-and-balance.com.* July 2009. <http://www.dizziness-and-balance.com/disorders/bppv>

Hain, Timothy C. "Otoliths." *Dizziness-and-balance.com.* April 2010. <http://www.dizziness-and-balance.com/disorders/bppv/otoliths. html>

Hain, Timothy C. "Postural, Vestibulospinal and Vestibulocollic Reflexes." *Dizziness-and-balance.com.* June 2009. <http://www.dizziness-and-balance.com/anatomy/vspine.htm>

Marieb, Elaine N., Mallatt, Jon, and Wilhelm, Patricia B. "The Ear: Hearing and Equilibrium." *Human Anatomy.* Fourth Edition. Chapter 16: 467-479. San Francisco: Pearson Benjamin Cummings, 2005. Print.

Mayo Clinic Staff. "Benign paroxysmal positional vertigo (BPPV)." *MayoClinic.com.* May 2008.
<http://www.mayoclinic.com/health/bppv>

Mayo Clinic. "Balance Problems.Types."*MayoClinic.com.* N.d. Retrieved August 2010.
<http://www.mayoclinic.org/balance-problems/types.html>

National Dizzy and Balance Center (NDBC) "Videonystagmography (VNG) Testing." N.d. Retrieved August 2010.
<http://www.stopdizziness.com/services-vng>

Swenson, Rand. "Vestibular System." *Review of Clinical and Functional Neuroscience.* Chapter 7E. Online version Dartmouth Medical School. January 2006.
<http://www.dartmouth.edu/~rswenson/NeuroSci/chapter-7E/vestibular-system>

Vestibular Disorders Association (VEDA).
"Electronystagmography (ENG)." August 2010.
<www.vestibular.org/vestibular-disorders/diagnostic-tests/eng>

Vestibular Disorders Association (VEDA). Balance: "Sensory Input." June 2010.
<http://www.vestibular.org/balance/sensory-input>

WebMD. "Electronystagmogram (ENG)." July 2010.
<http://www.webmd.com/brain/electronystagmogram-eng>

REFERENCES ARRANGED BY CHAPTER

Chapter 21 - Regaining Balance

Hain, Timothy C. "Vestibular Rehabilitation Therapy (VRT)." *Dizziness-and-balance.com.* November 2009. <http://www.dizziness-and-balance.com/treatment/rehab.html>

Mayo Clinic. "Balance Problems.Types." *MayoClinic.com.* n.d. Retrieved August 2010. <www.mayoclinic.org/balance-problems/types.html>

Vestibular Disorder Association (VEDA). "Vestibular Rehabilitation Therapy (VRT)." November 2010. <http://www.vestibular.org/treatment/ vestibular-rehabilitation>

Chapter 22 - Sudden Sensory Neural Hearing Loss (SSHL)

Bauman, Neil. "Sudden Sensorineural Hearing Loss (SSHL)." *Center for Hearing Loss Help.* June 2007. <http://www.hearinglosshelp.com/articles/suddenhearingloss>

Mathur, Neeraj, N and Carr, Michele M. "Inner Ear, Sudden Hearing Loss." *eMedicine Otolaryngology and Facial Plastic Surgery.* February 2009. <http://emedicine.medscape.com/article/856313-overview>

ScienceDaily. "Evidence Lacking to Guide Treatment for Sudden Hearing Loss." 20 June 2007. <www.sciencedaily.com/releases/2007/06/070618164138.htm>

National Institute on Deafness and Other Communication Disorders."Sudden Deafness." March 2003. <http://www.nidcd.nih.gov/health/hearing/sudden>

Chapter 23 - Ménière's Disease

Hain, Timothy C. "Ménière's Disease." *Dizziness-and-balance.com*. January 2010
<http://www.dizziness-and-balance.com/menieres.html>

Lundquist, PG. Abstract: "Aspects on Endolymphatic Sac Morphology and Function." September 16 1976. *PubMed.gov*.
<http://www.ncbi.nlm.nih.gov/pubmed/990076/aspects-on-endolymphatic-sac>

Mayo Clinic Staff. "Ménière's disease." *MayoClinic.com*. June 2010.
<http://mayoclinic.com/health/menieres-disease>

Ménière's Disease Information Center: "Symptoms. Cause.Treatment. Diagnosis." N.d. Retrieved March 2010.
<http://www.menieresinfo.com>

"Meniett Device." January 2006. (Air pulse generator).
<http://www.meniett.com/device.html>

National Dizzy and Balance Center. "Videonystagmography (VNG) Testing." N.d. Retrieved August 2010.
<http://www.stopdizziness.com/services-vng>

National Institute on Deafness and Other Communication Disorders. "Ménière's Disease." July 2010.
<www.nidcd.nih.gov/health/balance/meniere.html>

Paparella Otopathology Laboratory, University of Minnesota. "Ménière's Disease." N.d. Retrieved April 2011.
<http://www.otopathology.com/meniere.htm>

REFERENCES ARRANGED BY CHAPTER

Pray, W. Steven and Pray, Joshua J. "Ménière's Disease." *U.S. Pharmacist.* July 2005. 19-24. Print.

Salt, Alec N. "A Pictorial Guide to the Cochlear Fluids." *Cochlear Fluids Research Laboratory.* Washington University, St. Louis. N.d. Retrieved March 2010.
<http://oto2.wustl.edu/cochlea/intro1.html>

Vestibular Disorders Association (VEDA). "Electronystagmography (ENG)." August 2010.
<http://www.vestibular.org/vestibular-disorders/diagnostic-tests/eng>

Chapter 24 - Tinnitus

Bauman, Neil. "Musical Ear Syndrome." *Center for Hearing Loss Help.* January 2005.
<http://www.hearinglosshelp.com/articles/mes>

Calford, Michael B and Parsons, Carl H. "Abnormal Brain Activity in an Animal Model: Closing the Loop on Tinnitus. "*Tinnitus Today.* April 2008. 13, 22. Print.

Hain, Timothy C. "Tinnitus."*Dizziness-and-balance.com.*November 2010.
<http://www.dizziness-and-balance.com/disorders/tinnitus>

Holt, Avril Genene. "Gene Expression, A Clue to Turning Off Tinnitus." *Tinnitus Today.* December 2006. 17-19. Print.

Kaltenbach, James A. Abstract: "The Dorsal Cochlear Nucleus as a Participant in the Auditory, Attentional and Emotional Components of

Tinnitus." 15 February 2006. *PubMed.gov.*
<http://www.ncbi.nlm.nih.gov/pubmed/16469461>

Kaltenbach, James A. Abstract: "Summary of Evidence Pointing to a Role of the Dorsal Cochlear Nucleus in the Etiology of Tinnitus." December 2006. *PubMed.gov.*
<http://www.ncbi.nlm.nih.gov/pubmed/17114138>

Mayo Clinic Staff. "Tinnitus." *MayoClinic.com.* July 2010.
<http://www.mayoclinic.com/health/tinnitus/DS00365>

Melcher, Jennifer. "Brain Imaging in People with Tinnitus." *Tinnitus Today.* March 2007. 19. Print.

Chapter 25 - Tinnitus Types and the Importance of Medical Evaluation

Brantberg, Krister. Abstract: "Paroxysmal Staccato Tinnitus: a Carbamazepine responsive Hyperactivity Dysfunction Symptom of the Eighth Cranial Nerve." 23 September 2009. *Journal of Neurology, Neurosurgery & Psychiatry.*
<http://jnnp.bmj.com/content/81/4/451>

Drugwatch.com. "Drug Side Effects:Tinnitus." April 2011.
<http://www.drugwatch.com/side-effects > (click tinnitus).

Johnson, Marsha A. "Pulsatile Tinnitus Brief."
Tinnitus-audiology.com. Compiled April 1999.
<http://www.tinnitus-audiology.com/pulsatile>

REFERENCES ARRANGED BY CHAPTER

Lanska, Douglas J. Clinical Summary: "Subjective Tinnitus." *Medlink.com*. February 2011. <http://www.medlink.com/mlt000v2>

Letters to the Editor. "Tangled Arteries and Veins and Pulsatile Tinnitus." *Tinnitus Today*. December 2007:6. Print.

Shields, Gordon and Quinn, Francis B. "Tinnitus."(Objective Tinnitus). *Grand Rounds Presentation, UTMB, Department of Otolaryngology*. January 2003. <http://www.utmb.edu/otoref/grnds/Tinnitus-030122.html>

Shore, Susan E. "Roadmap to a Cure: Somatic Tinnitus." *Tinnitus Today*. March 2007. 8-9. Print.

Shore, Susan, Zhou Jianxun, and Koehler Seth. "Neural Mechanisms Underlying Somatic Tinnitus." 13 October 2008. *PubMed Central*. <http://www.ncbi.nlm.nih.gov/pmc/articles/PMC2566901/2008>

Chapter 26 - Tinnitus Management Basics

Author's Personal notes: Norman Berlinger, MD; Paparella Ear, Head and Neck Institute. 2009 Tinnitus Lecture at Marlys Soderberg Ménière's and Tinnitus Support Group, Minneapolis, MN.

Chapter 27 - Professional Tinnitus Management

American Hospital Formulary System (AHFS). "Benzodiazepines: General Statement." *AHFS Drug Information 2006*. 28:24.08. 2459-

67. Print. American Society of Health-System Pharmacists.

Ashton, Heather. "Benzodiazepines: How They Work and How to Withdraw." (Ashton Manual). *Benzo.org.uk.* August 2002. <www.benzo.org.uk/manual>

Bauman, Neil. "Neuromonics Tinnitus Treatment: Is It for Real?" *Center For Hearing Loss Help.* May 2009. <http://www.hearinglosshelp.com/articles/neuromonics>

FAQs: "Neuromonics Tinnitus Treatment: Frequently Asked Questions." N.d. Retrieved July 2010. *Neuromonics Inc.* <http://www.neuromonics.com/patient/treatment/faq.aspx>

Hain, Timothy C. "Tinnitus: Treatment." *Dizziness-and-balance.com.* November 2010. <http://www.dizziness-and-balance.com/disorders/tinnitus>

Hazell, Jonathan. "Tinnitus Retraining Therapy: Guidelines and Exercises for Patients." *The Tinnitus and Hyperacusis Site.* N.d. Retrieved June 2010. <http://www.tinnitus.org/home/frame/guidelines>

Highland, James. "Ultrasonic Treatment for Tinnitus." *eHow.com.* N.d. Retrieved June 2010. <http://www.ehow.com/ultrasonic-treatment-tinnitus>

Jastreboff, Pawel J. "Outline of TRT and Theoretical Basis of Approaches." *Tinnitus and Hyperacusis Center.* Emery University. May 1998. <http://www.tinnitus-pjj.com/approaches.html>

REFERENCES ARRANGED BY CHAPTER

Keate Barry. "Tinnitus Masking." *Quiet Times.* May 2004.
<http://www.tinnitusformula.com/qtimes/2004/05/mask.aspx>

Marcondes, Renata, Fregni, Felipe, and Pascual-Leone, Alvaro. Abstract. "Tinnitus and Brain Activation: Insights from Transcranial Magnetic Stimulation." April 2006. *PubMed.gov.*
<http://www.ncbi.nlm.nih.gov/pubmed/16696357>

Nagler, Stephen M. "Tinnitus Retraining Therapy (TRT)." *Dr. Nagler's Tinnitus Site.* N.d. Retrieved June 2010.
<http://home.comcast.net/~nagler/trt/html>

National Association of Cognitive-Behavioral Therapists. "Cognitive Behavioral Therapy." *NACBT Online Headquarters.* April 2007.
<htpp://www.nacbt.org/whatiscbt.html>

Netherlands Pharmacovigilance Centre Lareb. "SSRIs and tinnitus." *LAREB.NL.* November 2005.
<www.lareb.nl/documents/ssri>

Otis, James and Fudin Jeffrey. "Dependence, Tolerance, Addiction and Pseudoaddiction." (from article: Use of Long-Acting Opioids for the Management of Chronic Pain. *U.S. Pharmacist.* Supplement March 2005 edition. 9-10. Print.

Pittman, Genevra. "Magnetic Therapy May Not Relieve Ringing in the Ears." *Reuters Health.* April 22, 2013.
<http://www.reuters.com/article/2013/04/22/us-magnetic-therapy-idUSBRE93L14120130422>

Press Release. "New PSTR Treatment for Tinnitus Introduced at New York Academy of Medicine Symposium. February 2004.
<http://www.tinnituscare.net/news.html>

Robinson, Shannon, K. Abstract: "Antidepressants for Treatment of Tinnitus." October 2007. *PubMed.gov.*
<http://www.ncbi.nlm.nih.gov/pubmed/17956790>

Sandlin, Robert E. and Olsson, M.A. "Tinnitus: It Has a Certain Ring to it." *AudiologyOnline.* October 2000.
<http://www.audiologyonline.com/articles/tinnitus-it-has-a   certain-ring-to-it>

UCSF Medical Center: "Neuromonics." October 2010.
<http://www.ucsfhealth.org./neuromonics>

Chapter 28 - Excessive Noise Sensitivity: Recruitment and Hyperacusis

Bauman, Neil. "Recruitment from Hearing Loss Explained." *Center For Hearing Loss Help.* June 2001.
<http://www.hearinglosshelp.com/articles/recruitment>

Hain, Timothy C. "Hyperacusis." *Dizziness-and-balance.com.*
January 2008.
<http://www.dizziness-and-balance.com/disorders/hyperacusis.htm>

Hyperacusis Network. "Hyperacusis or Recruitment?" N.d. Retrieved November 2008.
<http://www.hyperacusis.net/hyperacusis/
hyperacusis+or+recruitment>

Hyperacusis Network. "What is Hyperacusis? What Can Be Done?" N.d. Retrieved November 2008.

<http://www.hyperacusis.net/hyperacusis/what+is+hyperacusis>
<http://www.hyperacusis.net/hyperacusis/what+can+be+done>

Hyperacusis Network. "Pink Noise." N.d. Retrieved November 2008.
<http://www.hyperacusis.net/hyperacusis/white+noisepink+noise>

Johnson, Marsha. Johnson Articles: "Distinguishing between Cochlear Hyperacusis and Vestibular Hyperacusis." *Tinnitus-audiology.com.* N.d. Retrieved November 2008.
<http://www.tinnitus-audiology.com/Cochlear>

Vestibular Disorders Association (VEDA. "Vestibular Hyperacusis."vMay 2010.
<http://www.vestibular.org/vestibular-hyperacusis>

Chapter 29 - Authorized to Buy a Hearing Aid and My First Hearing Aid Class

Ross, Mark. "Feedback Cancellation Systems and Open-Ear Hearing Aid Fitting." *Hearingresearch.org.* July 2006.
<http://www.hearingresearch.org/Dr.Ross/Feedback-Cancellation>

Chapter 30 - Hearing Aid Types and Styles

Consumer's Guide to Hearing Aids. 2009. Print.
<http://www.theconsumersguides.com/hearing-aids>

National Institute on Deafness and Other Communication Disorders. "Hearing Aids: Are there Different Styles of Hearing Aids? April 2007.
<http://www.nidcd.nih.gov/health/hearing/hearingaid.asp>

North Carolina, Hearing Loss Association of. "Direct Audio Input (DAI) Definition." N.d. Retrieved August 2010.
<http://www.nchearingloss.org/dai>

Extended-wear Hearing Device: "What is Lyric Hearing? *InSound Medical, Inc.* N.d. Retrieved August 2010.
<http://www.lyrichearing.com/what-is-lyric-hearing-aid/faq>

Invisible-In-The Canal (IIC) Hearing Aids: Starkey OtoLens. *Starkey Laboratories, Inc.* N.d. Retrieved September 2010.
<http://www.strakey.com/products/hearing-instrument/soundlens>

Chapter 31 - Hearing Instrument Technology

American Speech-Language-Hearing Association. "Hearing Aids." (Types of technology; features). N.d. Retrieved January 2009.
<http://www.asha.org/public/hearing/hearing-aids>

Calkins, Kelly C. "Understanding Hearing Aid Terms."December 2007.
<http://www.submityourarticle.com/articles/kelly-calkins/hearing-aid-terms>

Clark, Lynda. "What is the Optimum Number of Hearing Aid Channels?" *AudiologyOnline. Ask the Expert.* 1 September 2006.
<http://www.audiologyonline.com/askexpert/What-is-optimum-number-of-hearing-aid-channels>

Cochlear Americas. "The Baha system." (Bone-conduction processor). September 2010.
<http://products.cochlearamericas.com/baha-sysytem>

REFERENCES ARRANGED BY CHAPTER

Cochlear Americas. "Baha for Children." (Softband). December 2009.
<http://products.cochlearamericas.com/baha-for-children>

Consumer's Guide to Hearing Aids 2009. Print.
<http://www.theconsumersguides.com/hearing-aids>

HearingAid Help.com. "Selecting a Digital Hearing Aid." January 2008.
<http://www.hearingaidhelp.com/selecting-digital-hearing-aids>

National Institute on Deafness and Other Communication Disorders. "Hearing Aids: Do All Hearing Aids Work the Same?" April 2007.
<http://www.nidcd.nih.gov/health/hearing/hearingaid.asp>

Deaf Access.org. "Bone Conductive Hearing Aids."N.d. Retrieved January 2011.
<http://www.deafaccess.org/bone-conductive-hearing-aids>

Royal National Institute for Deaf People (RNID). "Bone-conduction Hearing Aids. October 2000.
<www.clickhearing.com/pdf/bone-conduction-hearing-aid>

Chapter 32 - Buying a Hearing Aid: Practitioners, Regulations, Sales

American Board of Audiology (ABA). "What is ABA Certification?" N.d. Retrieved August 2010.
<http://www.americanboardofaudiology.org/faq/what-is-aba-certification>

American Speech-Language-Hearing Association (ASHA). "General Information About ASHA Certification." N.d. Retrieved December 2010.
<www.asha.org/AboutCertificationGenInfo>

Federal Trade Commission (FTC). "Sound Advice on Hearing Aids." September 2010.
<http://www.ftc.gov/bcp/edu/pubs/hea10.shtml>

National Board for Certification in Hearing Instrument Sciences (NBC-HIS). August 2008.
<http://www.nbc-his.com>

Chapter 33 - Buying a Hearing Aid: Balancing Trust and Caution

ESCO. "Hearing Aid Insurance." N.d. Retrieved January 2011.
<http://www.earserv.com/consumers/esco-coverage>

HearSource.com. Hearing Aid Sitemap: "Hearing Aid Programming Software. Video Tutorials. Remote Programming Support. N.d. Retrieved November 2010.
<http://www.hearsource.com/programming-software>
<http://www.<http://www.hearsource.com/video-tutorials>
<http://www.hearsource.com/remote-programming-support>

Chapter 34 - Assistive listening devices (ALDs) and Applications

Aarts, Nancy L. "T-Coils: Getting the Most Out of Your Hearing Aid." *AudiologyOnline.* August 2004.
<http://www.audiologyonline.com/article/t-coils-getting-the most>

REFERENCES ARRANGED BY CHAPTER

American Speech-Language-Hearing Association. "Hearing Aids and Cell Phones." a*sha.org* N.d. Retrieved May 2015. <http://www.asha.org/public/hearing/Hearing-Aids-and-Cell-Phones/>

Ampetronic. "Standard Compliant Hearing Loop Installations to Become Law in America." *ampetronic.com* December 2013. <http://www.ampetronic.com/Blog/americanhearinglooplaw>

Beck, Douglas L. "T-coils: Beyond the Telephone."*AudiologyOnline.* October 2006. <http://www.audiologyonline.com/articles/t-coils-beyond-the-telephone>

Hain, Timothy C. and Rudisill, Heather. "Loop Systems and Telecoils for Hearing Aids." *Dizziness-and-balance.com.* August 2010. <http://www.dizziness-and-balance.com/hearing-aids/tcoil>

Hammond, Monique E. "Tips on Vetting Hearing Loop Installers." *moniquehammond.com* July 2014. <http://moniquehammond.com/tips-vetting-hearing-loop-installers/>

Harris Communications. "Products for Deaf and Hard-of-Hearing People." Catalog. Print. <http://www.harriscomm.com>

Minnesota, State of, Dept. of Human Services." Fact sheet: Cell phones for people with hearing aids. January 2011. <http://www.dhs.state.mn.us/deaf-and-hard-of-hearing/cell-phone-factsheet>

North Carolina, Hearing Loss Association of. "Direct Audio Input (DAI) Definition."N.d. Retrieved August 2010.
<http://www.nchearingloss.org/dai>

Ross, Mark. "More on Telecoils." *Hearing Loss Web*. N.d. Retrieved January 2009.
<http://www.hearinglossweb.com/tech/ha/conv/tcoil/ross>

Williams Sound. "Assistive Listening Solutions." Catalog. Print.
<http://www.williamssound.com>

Chapter 35 - American Sign Language (ASL) and Speech Reading

Bauman, Neil. "Speechreading (Lip-reading)." *Center for Hearing Loss Help*. March 2000.
<http://www.hearinglosshelp.com/articles/speechreading>

Berke, Jamie. "Lipreading (or Speechreading)." *About.com Deafness*. April 2014.
<http://deafness.about.com/cs/communication/a/lipreading.htm>

Chapter 37 - Middle Ear Implants (MEIs)

Anderson, Liz. "The Esteem Hearing Implant." *AudiologyOnline* July 2014
<http://www.audiologyonline.com/articles/the-esteem-middle-ear-implant-12780>

Ear Institute of Chicago. "Vibrant Soundbridge." N.d. Retrieved April 2015.(Semi-implant MEI).

REFERENCES ARRANGED BY CHAPTER

<www.chicagoear.com/implantable/vibrant-soundbridge>

FDA Medical Devices. "Esteem Implantable Hearing System." June 2010. (Full-implant MEI).
<http://www.fda.gov/MedicalDevices/esteem>

Frenzel, H., Hanke, F., Beltrame, M., Steffen, A., Schönweiler, R., Wollenberg, B. Abstract: "Application of the Vibrant Soundbridge to Unilateral Osseous Atresia Cases." January 2009. *PubMed.gov.*
<http://www.ncbi.nlm.nih.gov/pubmed/19117311>

Video. "How the Vibrant Soundbridge Works." *medel.com* N.d. Retrieved April 2015
<http://www.medel.com/us/how-the-vibrant-soundbridge-works>

Chapter 38 - Cochlear Implants and Auditory Brainstem Implant

Advanced Bionics. "HiRes 90K Implant Family." *advancedbionics. com* N.d. Retrieved February 2015.
<http://www.advancedbionics.com/com/en/products/hires_90k_implant.html>

Carver, Courtney L."Cochlear Implant Mapping." *Hearing Loss Magazine* July/August 2007.10-13. Print.

Cochlear. "The Nucleus 6 Sound Processor." *cochlear.com* N.d. Retrieved March 2015.
<http://www.cochlear.com/wps/wcm/connect/us/home/treatment-options-for-hearing-loss/cochlear-implants/nucleus-6-features>

Cochlear. "Cochlear Hybrid Hearing Solution." *cochlear.com* N.d. Retrieved February 2015.
<http://www.cochlear.com/wps/wcm/connect/us/home/N6hybrid/index.html>

Cochlear Implant HELP. "Recalls." *cochlearimplanthelp.com* N.d. Retrieved March 2015.
<http://cochlearimplanthelp.com/journey/choosing-a-cochlear-implant/cochlear-implant-problems/recalls/>

Ear Surgery Information Center. "Cochlear Implants." *earsurgery.org* N.d. Retrieved March 2015.
<http://www.earsurgery.org/surgery/cochlear-implants/>

MED-EL. "RONDO Single-Unit Processor for Cochlear Implants." *medel.com* N.d. Retrieved January 2015.
<http://www.medel.com/us/rondo>

MED-EL. "Auditory Brainstem Implant (ABI)." *medel.com* N.d. Retrieved March 2015.
<http://www.medel.com/maestro-components-abi/>

National Association of the Deaf (NAD). "Cochlear Implants: NAD Position Statement on Cochlear Implants. October 2000.
<http://www.nad.org/cochlear-implants>

National Institute on Deafness and Other Communication Disorders. "Quick Statistics." June 2010.
<http://www.nidcd.nih.gov/health/statistics/quick>

National Institute on Deafness and Other Communication Disorders. "Cochlear Implants." May 2007.
<http//www.nidcd.nih.gov/health/hearing/coch.asp>

Powerhouse Museum. "Cochlear Implant: Volta's Crazy Experiments." N.d. Retrieved March 2009.
<http://www.powerhousemuseum.com/hsc/cochlear/history/Volta>

Chapter 39 - Bone-Conduction Implants

Bauman, Neil. "What are CROS and Bi-Cros Hearing Aids?" *Hearing Loss Help*. March 2007.
<http://hearinglosshelp.com/weblog/what-are-cros-hearing-aids>

Cochlear."Baha 4 Connect System." *cochlear.com* N.d. Retrieved March 2015.
<http://www.cochlear.com/wps/wcm/connect/au/home/discover/baha-bone-conduction-implants/baha-connect-system>

Cochlear. "Baha 4 Attract System." *cochlear.com*. N.d. Retrieved March 2015.
<http://www.cochlear.com/wps/wcm/connect/us/for-professionals/products/baha/products/baha-attract-system>

Hearing Loss Association of North Carolina. "CROS and BICROS Definition." N.d. Retrieved August 2015 *www.nchearingloss.org*
< http://www.nchearingloss.org/bicros.htm>

MED-EL. "How the BONEBRIDGE Works – YouTube." *medel.com* N.d. Retrieved May 2015.
<www.youtube.com/watch?v=Wfc3ymniURI>

Sinopoli, Terri. "Oticon Medical: Introduction to the Ponto Bone An-chored System." May 8, 2012. *AudiologyOnline*
<http://www.audiologyonline.com/articles/oticon-medical-introduc-tion-to-ponto-6580>

Sophono. "Abutment Free Magnetic Bone Conduction Hearing De-vice." *sophono.com* N.d. Retrieved April 2015.
<https://sophono.com/professionals/bone-conduction-hearing-de-vice/>

Maryland, University of, Medical Center. "Bone-anchored Devices." July 2014.
<http://umm.edu/programs/hearing/services/bone-anchored-devices>

Chapter 40 - Feelings and Emotions

Changing Minds.org. "The Kübler-Ross Grief Cycle." N.d. Retrieved April 2009.
<http://changingminds.org/kubler-ross-grief-cycle>

Quote Garden. Attitude Quotes by Winston Churchill and
   Hubert H. Humphrey.
    <www.quotegarden.com/attitude>

Chapter 43 - Future Outlook

Brainy Quote. Quote by Dr. Martin Luther King Jr.

GLOSSARY - INDEX

GLOSSARY - INDEX

ABR: auditory brainstem response test; same as BAER.
(See chapter 12   P. 61)

acoustic feedback (hearing aids): squealing noise resulting from the recycling of leaked, already amplified sound through the hearing instrument.
(See chapter 29   P. 227)

ALD: assistive listening device; device other than a hearing aid that helps those with hearing loss hear better.
(See chapter 34   P. 271)

air conduction: sound wave propagation through the air from the outer to the inner ear.
(See chapter 12, 30   P. 59, 234)

amplifier: electronic device that adds power (gain) to an electrical signal.
(See chapters 2, 31   *P. 7, 244)

analog sound: sound signal in the form of a continuous wave.
(See chapter 31, 34   P. 243, 275)

antidepressants: classes of medications used primarily to relieve depression.
(See chapter 27   P. 207)

antioxidants: chemicals which neutralize free radicals that cause oxidative damage to tissues and organs.
(See chapter 16   P. 105)

anvil: incus; second (middle) bone of the middle-ear ossicle chain.
(See chapter 11   P. 46)

ASHA: American-Speech-Language-Hearing Association.
(See chapter 13, 14, 32   P. 75, 79, 256)

ATA: American Tinnitus Association.
(See chapter 24   P. 160)

audiogram: record depicting the results of hearing tests.
(See chapter 12, 13   P. 55, 69)

audiologist: a health care professional specialized in problems related to hearing and balance.
(See chapter 12, 32   P. 55, 255)

auricle: pinna; external, visible part of the ear.
(See chapter 11   P. 44)

autoimmune reaction: condition where the body's immune system attacks parts of itself.
(See chapter 15, 22   P. 44, 89)

BAHA: bone anchored hearing aid; a hearing system that transmits sound vibrations to the inner ear by means of an implanted titanium stud.
(See chapter 39   P. 307)

BAER test: brainstem auditory evoked response; same as ABR.
(See chapter 12   P. 62)

balance retraining: exercises to help rebuild strength and re-learn coordination skills for maintaining equilibrium.
(See chapters 6, 21   P. 21, 134)

BBPV: benign paroxysmal positional vertigo; an inner-ear condition that causes dizziness.
(See chapter 4, 20   P. 14, 128)

benign paroxysmal positional vertigo: BPPV; an inner-ear condition that causes dizziness.
(See chapter 4, 20   P. 14, 128)

benzodiazepines or benzos: class of medications used mostly for their tranquilizing and anti-anxiety effect; also stabilize the vestibular (balance) system.
(See chapter 27   P. 201)

bone anchored hearing aid: BAHA; a hearing system that transmits sound vibrations to the inner ear by means of an implanted titanium stud.
(See chapter 39   P. 307)

bone conduction: transmission of sound vibrations to the cochlea by the skull and jaw bones.
(See chapter 12   P. 60)

BTE: behind-the-ear hearing aid.
(See chapter 30   P. 235)

CART: Communication Access Real time Translation. A system where a person using court reporting software types in the discussion during a meeting. The text is then projected onto a screen using an LCD projector.
(See chapter 34   P. 276)

CBT: cognitive-behavioral therapy; a psychotherapy technique that teaches how to change or adjust the thinking process on a particular issue.
(See chapter 27   P. 192)

cerumen: earwax.
(See chapter 11, 12   P. 44, 67)

CI: cochlear implant; implanted, electronic hearing system; gives a sense of sound to people who are deaf or severely hard of hearing.
(See chapter 38   P. 297)

CIC: completely-in-canal hearing aid; hardly visible.
(See chapter 30   P. 240)

cochlear duct: snail-shaped tube housing the hearing cells of the inner ear.
(See chapter 11   P. 48)

cochlear implant: CI; implanted, electronic hearing system; gives a sense of sound to people who are deaf or severely hard of hearing.
(See chapter 38   P. 297)

cognitive-behavioral therapy: CBT; a psychotherapy technique that teaches how to change or adjust the thinking process on a particular issue.
(See chapter 27   P. 192)

compression: hearing aid sound-adjusting process; keeps annoying or harmful sounds from becoming too loud.
(See chapter 31   P. 248)

conductive hearing loss: hearing loss related to outer and/or middle ear problems.
(See chapter 12, 31, 39   P. 63, 251, 307)

corticosteroids: group of medications that lower inflammation and suppress the immune system.
(See chapter 22, 23   P. 142, 153)

dB: decibel; audiology unit for measuring sound volume or intensity (loudness).
(See chapter 13, 14   P. 73, 79)

DCN: dorsal cochlear nucleus; brainstem relay for electrical sound signals; suspected of playing a role in tinnitus.
(See chapter 24, 25   P. 159, 165)

decibel: dB; audiology unit for measuring sound volume or intensity (loudness).
(See chapter 13, 14   P. 73, 79)

digital sound: electrical sound signal that has been "digitized," or organized into series of 1s and 0s.
(See chapter 31   P. 245)

diuretic, or water pill: medication that helps the body eliminate excess water.
(See chapter 6, 23   P. 27, 152)

earwax: also called cerumen
(See chapter 11, 12   P. 44, 67)

eardrum: tympanic membrane; separates the outer and middle ear.
(See chapter 11, 12, P. 45, 58)

eighth cranial nerve: made of the cochlear and vestibular nerves; also called vestibulo-cochlear nerve.
(See chapter 11, 19 P. 54, 123)

endolymph: liquid that fills the membranous labyrinth of the inner ear.
(See chapter 11, 20 P. 48, 127)

ENT: ear, nose, and throat; a doctor who specializes in these areas of the body.
(See chapter 6, 25 P. 15, 162)

equilibrium tripod: conveys the teamwork of three systems to maintain balance: ear, eyes, and body sensors.
(See chapter 20 P. 125)

eustachian canal, or tube: connects the middle ear to the throat; also called pharyngotympanic tube.
(See chapter 11, 25 P. 45, 168)

external ear: also called the outer ear; made of the pinna (visible part) and the external ear canal.
(See chapter 11 P. 44)

FDA: U.S. Food and Drug Administration; enforces regulations on hearing aid manufacture and sale.
(See chapter 17, 32 P. 116, 258)

hearing aid (instrument): electronic device for adjusting sound signals to help people with hearing loss hear more distinctly.
(See chapter 30, 31, 32   P. 233, 243, 255)

hearing instrument dispenser: HID; state authorized practitioner involved with hearing aid fitting and sales.
(See chapter 32   P. 256)

hearing loss: amount of hearing decline—expressed in decibels—registered over a set spectrum of test frequencies.
(See chapter 12, 13, 14, 15, 16   P. 55, 69, 79, 85, 95)

hearing loss classification: system for rating the degree of hearing loss based on decibel losses.
(See chapter 14   P. 80)

HID: hearing instrument dispenser; state authorized practitioner involved with hearing aid fitting and sale.
(See chapter 32   P. 256)

hyperacusis: a condition where everyday sounds appear to be way too loud.
(See chapter 7, 28   P. 27, 211)

idiopathic: without a known cause.
(See chapter 20, 22, 23   P. 128, 140, 149)

IIC: invisible-in-the-canal hearing aid.
(See chapter 30   P. 241)

incus: anvil; second (middle) bone of the middle-ear ossicle chain.
(See chapter 11   P. 46)

inner ear: also called labyrinth; portion of the ear involved with hearing and balance.
(See chapter 11 P. 47)

IR: infrared; method for transmitting sound signals wirelessly from a source to a receiver.
(See chapter 34 P. 273)

ITC: in-the-canal hearing aid.
(See chapter 30 P. 240)

ITE: in-the-ear hearing aid; fills the concha, or bowl, of the outer ear.
(See chapter 30 P. 238)

labyrinth: means "maze;" collective name for the bony and membranous structures of the inner ear.
(See chapter 11 P. 47)

labyrinthitis: infection of the inner ear; usually viral.
(See chapter 4 P. 15)

looping: method of using electromagnetic energy to provide clearer sound signals to devices equipped with a T-coil.
(See chapter 34 P. 280)

loudspeaker: called "receiver" in hearing aids; converts an electrical signal back into a sound wave
(See chapter 31 P. 238)

malleus: hammer; first bone of the middle-ear ossicle chain; attaches to eardrum.
(See chapter 11 P. 46)

masking (hearing tests): method for "isolating" the test-ear during hearing tests by feeding static noise to the non-test ear.
(See chapter 12, 13   P. 60, 78)

masking (tinnitus): technique for covering up internal sounds—tinnitus—with external sounds, or masking sounds.
(See chapter 27   P. 187)

measles: contagious viral disease that can lead to hearing loss and deafness.
(See chapter 15   P. 91)

MedWatch: FDA's safety and adverse events reporting program.
(See chapter 17   P. 116)

Ménière's disease: condition considered to be caused by inner-ear endolymph pressure increases.
(See chapter 15, 23   P. 87, 145)

microphone: electronic device; converts captured sound waves into electrical signals.
(See chapter 31   P. 244)

middle ear: air-filled chamber starting at the eardrum and extending to the inner ear.
(See chapter 11   P. 45)

MRI: magnetic resonance imaging; diagnostic method; visualizes structures of the human body without X-rays.
(See chapter 6, 18   P. 23, 119)

mumps: contagious viral disease that can lead to hearing loss and deafness.
(See chapter 15   P. 91)

Neuromonics: professionally guided method for treating tinnitus.
(See chapter 27   P. 193)

NIHL: noise-induced hearing loss.
(See chapter 16   P. 95)

NIOSH: National Institute for Occupational Safety and Health.
(See chapter 16   P. 101)

NRR: noise reduction rating for earplugs.
(See chapter 16   P. 104)

noise-induced hearing loss: NIHL
(See chapter 16   P. 95)

nystagmus: involuntary, rapid eye movements.
(See chapter 5, 23   P. 19, 150)

OAE: otoacoustic emissions; hearing test evaluating cochlear hair cell function.
(See chapter 12   P. 62)

objective tinnitus: ear noises that can be detected by the doctor or audiologist.
(See chapter 25   P. 166)

organ of Corti: spiral of tuned hair cells located in the cochlear duct of the inner ear.
(See chapter 11   P. 49)

OSHA: occupational safety and health administration; federal regulatory agency.
(See chapter 16…P. 101)

ossicles: three small bones located in the middle ear.
(See chapter 11   P. 46)

otoconia: small crystals, referred to as ear rocks; important for maintaining balance.
(See chapter 4, 20   P. 14, 127)

otosclerosis: middle ear condition; stapes ossicle becomes fixed; leads to hearing loss.
(See chapter 12, 15   P. 58, 88)

ototoxic substance: any chemical that damages the hearing and/or balance structures of the inner ear.
(See chapter 17   P. 109)

oval window: upper membrane-covered opening between the middle and the inner ear.
(See chapter 11   P. 45)

perilymph: fluid that surrounds the inner ear structures of the membranous labyrinth.
(See chapter 11   P. 48)

pink noise: sound blend of random frequencies; helpful in the treatment of hyperacusis.
(See chapter 28   P. 217)

pinna: auricle; external, visible part of the ear.
(See chapter 11   P. 44)

pitch: perceived frequency of a sound.
(See chapter 13   P. 70)

prednisone: corticosteroid medication; has anti-inflammatory and immune-suppression activities.
(See chapter 5   P. 22)

PSTR: phase-shift-tinnitus reduction; technique for canceling out tinnitus noise made of only one frequency.
(See chapter 27   P. 190)

PTA score: pure-tone average score; expresses the average dB hearing loss over 3 speech frequencies.
(See chapter 14   P. 80)

pulsatile tinnitus: ear noise with a rhythmic, pulsing quality; often detectable by clinician.
(See chapter 25   P. 166)

pure-tone audiometry: test procedure using pure, single frequency tones to evaluate hearing sensitivity.
(See chapter 12   P. 58)

real-ear measures: method for verifying actual hearing aid or T-coil sound output at the eardrum level.
(See chapter 29, 34   P. 226, 280)

receiver (hearing aid): hearing aid's loudspeaker; converts electrical signals back into sound waves.
(See chapter 31   P. 238)

recruitment: refers to a rapid sound intensity escalation as a consequence of hearing loss due to cochlear hair cell and/or nerve damage.
(See chapter 28   P. 211)

repetitive transcranial magnetic stimulation: rTMS; tinnitus treatment technique; not yet FDA approved.
(See chapter 27   P. 191)

RIC: receiver-in-canal hearing aid.
(See chapter 30   P. 238)

round window: lower membrane-covered opening between the middle and inner ear.
(See chapter 11   P. 45)

rTMS: repetitive transcranial magnetic stimulation; tinnitus treatment technique; not yet FDA approved.
(See chapter 27   P. 191)

saccule: inner ear otolith (ear rock) organ; important for balance.
(See chapter 11, 20   P. 48, 126)

semicircular ducts: three inner-ear, looped tubes housing balance motion-sensor cells.
(See chapter 11, 20   P. 48, 126)

sensorineural hearing loss: irreversible hearing loss due to cochlear cell and/or nerve damage.
(See chapter 12, 22   P. 63, 139)

somatic tinnitus: ear noises with a somatic, or body, connection.
(See chapter 25   P. 165)

sound processor: hearing aid circuitry for adjusting electrical signals. (See chapter 31, 37, 38, 39   P. 247, 295, 301, 308)

staccato tinnitus: ear noises that sound like popping popcorn or typewriter taps. (See chapter 25   P. 168)

stapedius muscle: middle ear muscle attaching to the stapes ossicle. (See chapter 11, 12   P. 47, 58)

stapes: stirrup; third bone of the middle ear ossicle chain. (See chapter 11   P. 46)

stereo: sound setting giving illusion of being surrounded by sounds and hearing them equally well on both ears. (See chapter 26, 39   P. 180, 282)

subjective tinnitus: ear or head noises only "heard" by patient; undetectable by doctor or audiologist. (See chapter 25   P. 161)

sudden sensorineural hearing loss: SSHL; hearing loss that happens over a period of three days or less. (See chapter 22   P. 139)

syphilis: venereal disease; can lead to hearing loss in the later stages of the disease. (See chapter 15   P. 92)

T-coil or **telecoil**; installed in hearing aids and other assistive listening devices for increased sound quality during telephone use and in looped environments. (See chapter 34   P. 275)

tensor tympani: middle ear muscle; attaches to the malleus, or hammer.
(See chapter 11   P. 47)

tinnitus: ear or head noises of different origins, types, and tones.
(See chapter 24, 25   P. 157, 161)

tinnitus masking: technique for covering up internal sounds—tinnitus—with external sounds, or masking sounds.
(See chapter 27   P. 187)

tinnitus retraining therapy (TRT): professionally guided tinnitus treatment technique for habituating the noise.
(See chapter 27   P. 193)

tumor: abnormal tissue growth; can be cancerous or benign.
(See chapter 15, 19   P. 92, 123)

tympanic membrane: eardrum; separates the outer and middle ear.
(See chapter 11, 12   P. 44, 57)

tympanometry: series of tests evaluating the function of the middle ear.
(See chapter 12   P. 57)

ultrasound: refers to sound frequencies above the normal human hearing range.
(See chapter 27   P. 191)

utricle: inner ear otolith (ear rock) organ; important for balance.
(See chapter 11, 20   P. 48, 126)

vascular: refers to blood vessels.
(See chapter 15, 25   P. 87, 209)

vestibular neuritis: inflammation of the vestibular (balance) nerve due to a viral infection; can cause severe dizziness and nausea.
(See chapter 4   P. 14)

vestibular rehabilitation: VRT; therapy exercises to rebuild strength and re-learn coordination skills for maintaining equilibrium
(See chapter 20   P. 134)

vestibule: part of the inner ear bony labyrinth; located roughly between the cochlea and the semicircular canals.
(See chapter 11, 20   P. 48, 126)

VCR: vestibulo-collic reflex; helps stabilize the head.
(See chapter 20   P. 130)

VOR: vestibulo-ocular reflex; keeps objects in focus as head moves.
(See chapter 20   P. 129)

VRT: vestibular rehabilitation; therapy exercises to rebuild strength and re-learn coordination skills for maintaining equilibrium
(See chapter 20   P. 134)

VSR: vestibulo-spinal reflex; automatically adjusts body posture for maintaining equilibrium.
(See chapter 20   P. 130)

white noise: sound blend made of all frequencies audible to the human ear; used to mask tinnitus noises.
(See chapter 26, 27   P. 178, 187)